CHAIR YOGA FOR SENIORS OVER 60

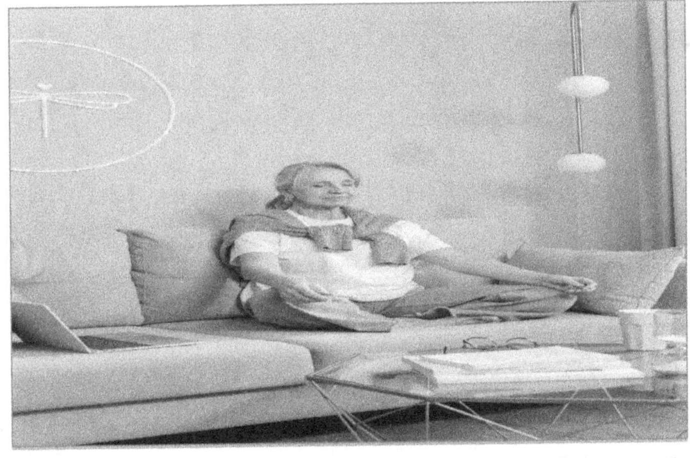

Achieve better balance, mobility, and quick flexibility with these simple, quick, and effective chair yoga exercises, plus 7days meal plan to improve your health

Anthony Howell

TABLE OF CONTENTS

Introduction

Discovering Chair Yoga: A Personal Journey

Exploring the Benefits of Chair Yoga

How This Book Can Guide You

Chapter 1: Getting Started with Chair Yoga

What is Chair Yoga?

The Importance of Chair Yoga for Seniors

Safety Precautions and Guidelines

Chapter 2: Gentle Chair Yoga Poses for Seniors of All Levels

Introduction to Gentle Chair Yoga Poses

Sitting stretches and breathing exercises

Mindful Movement Techniques for Seniors.

Chapter 3: Chair Yoga for Balance and Stability

Importance of Balance and Stability in Aging

Chair Yoga Poses for Improving Balance and Core Strength

Benefits of Chair Yoga for Improving Balance and Core Strength:

Progression Exercises for Improved Stability

Common problems and challenges with balance

How to overcome typical issues associated with balance

Chapter 4: Chair Yoga for Flexibility and Mobility

Improving Flexibility and Mobility with Chair Yoga

Chair Yoga: A Path to Greater Freedom.

Exploring Gentle Yoga Poses

Embrace the Journey

Gentle Stretching Routines to Improve Range of Motion

Techniques to relieve joint stiffness and pain

Chapter 5: Mindfulness and Stress Reduction

Effects of Mindfulness on the Brain and Body

Chair Yoga Techniques for Stress Relief

Practices for Promoting Inner Peace and Relaxation

Chapter 6: Chair Yoga for Specific Health Concerns

Adapting Chair Yoga to Common Health Conditions

Chair Yoga for Arthritis, Osteoporosis, And Diabetes

Pose and Modifications for Pain Relief and Rehabilitation

Chapter 7: 7-Day Chair Yoga Meal Plan

Day 1: Energizing Start

Day 2: Nourishing Nutrition

Day 3: Balanced bliss.

Day 4: Wholesome Delights.

Day 5: Flavored Feasts

Day 6: Energizing Eats

Day 7: Nourishing Nutrition

Conclusion: Embrace Wellness with Chair Yoga

Encouragement of Continued Practice and Growth

Introduction

As we age, it's critical to find methods to keep active and healthy. Many seniors find conventional yoga postures too difficult or hazardous, and some abandon the practice entirely. But there's another option: chair yoga. Chair yoga is a modified version of yoga in which a chair supports the body, making it safer and more accessible to elders.

Welcome to the world of chair yoga, a gentle and accessible practice created exclusively for adults over 60. In this introduction part, we welcome you to learn about the various advantages of chair yoga and how it may help you on your path to greater health and wellness.

Discovering Chair Yoga: A Personal Journey

Maria, my lovely aunt and mother's elder sister, has always been a source of strength in our family, but when she was faced with the enormous difficulty of coping with her husband's death, she felt confused and overwhelmed.

When I originally proposed chair yoga to Maria, she was skeptical. She thought she was too elderly to participate in yoga positions and discarded the concept entirely. However, I continued, gently explaining the advantages and assured her that chair yoga could be modified to meet her requirements.

Maria reluctantly decided to give it a try. With compassion and encouragement, I led her through easy chair yoga poses, emphasizing how the practice may benefit both her physical and mental health.

To my astonishment and happiness, Maria began to exhibit positive behaviour almost immediately. Her muscles relaxed, and she discovered the calm and tranquillity she had been looking for months. Maria's confidence rose as she practiced more, and she realized that age was no barrier to the advantages of yoga.

Maria was encouraged by her development and renewed Vigor, so she embraced chair yoga enthusiastically. She got enthusiastic about sharing her story with others, promoting the message that it's never too late to begin your road to health and fitness.

Exploring the Benefits of Chair Yoga

Chair yoga has several advantages for seniors, ranging from increased flexibility and mobility to decreased tension and anxiety. Its gentle, approachable character makes yoga appropriate for people of all fitness levels and physical abilities, allowing everyone to receive the benefits of this ancient practice.

Chair yoga is a safe and effective approach for seniors to get the benefits of yoga without requiring difficult positions. Using a chair as support, participants may easily engage in a range of motions and stretches that enhance flexibility, strength, and relaxation.

How This Book Can Guide You

In the pages that follow, we'll go deep into the realm of chair yoga, looking at a range of postures, methods, and sequences intended exclusively for seniors over 60. Drawing on Maria's journey and my own experiences as a yoga practitioner, I will walk you through each component of the practice, providing practical ideas, guidance, and support along the way.

So, let us discover together, the limitless possibilities of chair yoga and the tremendous influence it can have on our lives.

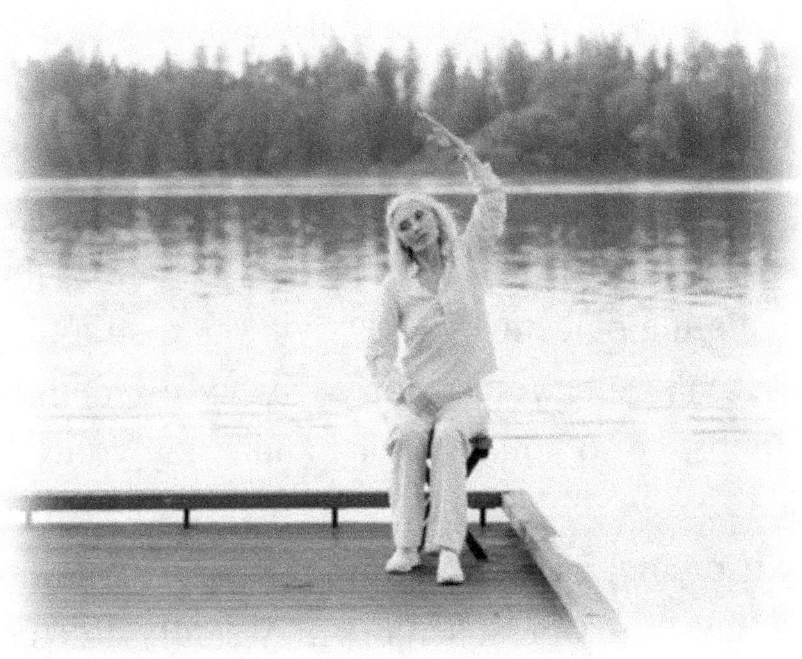

Chapter 1: Getting Started with Chair Yoga

If you're over 60 and searching for a mild, low-impact strategy to stay active and enhance your health, chair yoga might be the answer. Chair yoga is a modified version of yoga that is performed while sitting in a chair. This makes it ideal for people who have restricted movement or are uncomfortable with standing yoga positions. Creating a welcoming environment is a crucial element of beginning your chair yoga adventure. A location that is relaxing and appealing will allow you to relax and concentrate on your practice. Consider burning a candle or using a diffuser with a relaxing aroma like lavender or chamomile. You might either listen to relaxing music or find a quiet place to practice without distractions. Finally, make sure your chair yoga environment is safe and supportive so you can relax and enjoy your practice.

Safety is crucial in any workout practice, including chair yoga. While most seniors may safely do chair yoga, it's important to listen to your body and practice with mindfulness and awareness. If you have any current health ailments or concerns, contact your healthcare physician before beginning a chair yoga practice.

What is Chair Yoga?

Chair yoga is a moderate type of yoga that is done while sitting on a chair or using a chair for support. It is a modified form of traditional yoga, making it suitable for anyone who struggles with balance, movement, or getting up and down from the floor. Chair yoga combines several yoga postures, breathing exercises, and meditation techniques that are all designed to be practiced while sitting comfortably in a chair.

One of the primary advantages of chair yoga is its adaptability. It can be tailored to people of different ages and fitness levels, making it an ideal choice for elders, those recuperating from injuries, or anybody searching for a gentle method to enhance their physical and mental health.

Chair yoga has various advantages, including increased flexibility, strength, and balance. It helps to gently stretch and strengthen muscles, promote joint mobility, and improve posture—all without placing too much strain on the body. In addition, chair yoga can help reduce stress, anxiety, and sadness, increasing relaxation and general well-being.

The Importance of Chair Yoga for Seniors

Chair yoga benefits seniors' health and well-being in a variety of ways.

Accessibility: Chair yoga is a safe and accessible solution for seniors with mobility, balance, or other physical impairments. Seniors can still benefit from yoga by practicing while seated, without having to go up and down from the floor.

Physical Health: Chair yoga improves seniors' physical health by enhancing flexibility, strength, and balance. Gentle motions and stretches keep muscles and joints flexible and supple, lowering the chance of injury and increasing general mobility.

Mental Well-Being: In addition to its physical benefits, chair yoga promotes mental and emotional health. Seniors can reduce stress, worry, and depression by focusing on breath awareness and mindfulness, which promotes a sense of serenity and inner peace.

Social Connection: Chair yoga courses allow seniors to mingle and connect with others in a friendly and accepting setting. This sense of community can assist in alleviating feelings of loneliness and isolation by fostering a sense of belonging and companionship.

Overall, chair yoga is a gentle and effective approach for seniors to be active, healthy, and connected as they age. Seniors who incorporate chair yoga into their daily routine might experience increased physical and mental well-being, a higher quality of life, and a greater feeling of energy and joy.

Setting Up Your Space for Chair Yoga

Before you start your chair yoga practice, make sure you have a comfortable and appealing location where you can rest and focus. Here are some recommendations for preparing your environment for chair yoga:

Find a peaceful spot: Select a peaceful spot in your house where you will not be disturbed while practicing. Ideally, this place should be devoid of distractions and large enough to allow you to easily adjust your chair.

Choose a Sturdy Chair: Choose a chair that has a straight back and no arms. Avoid chairs with wheels or swivel bases, as they may not provide adequate stability during practice.

Use Props and Accessories: Gather any props or accessories you may require to aid your practice, such as cushions, blankets, and yoga blocks. These tools can make your practice more pleasant and accessible.

Set the Mood: Create a calm ambiance in your practice area by lowering the lights, playing gentle music, or burning candles or incense. This might help you stay grounded and focused during your practice.

Remove Shoes and Socks: Before beginning your practice, remove your shoes and socks to let your feet touch with the ground and maintain stability throughout your postures.

By carefully arranging your area, you may create a setting that promotes your chair yoga practice while also improving your entire experience.

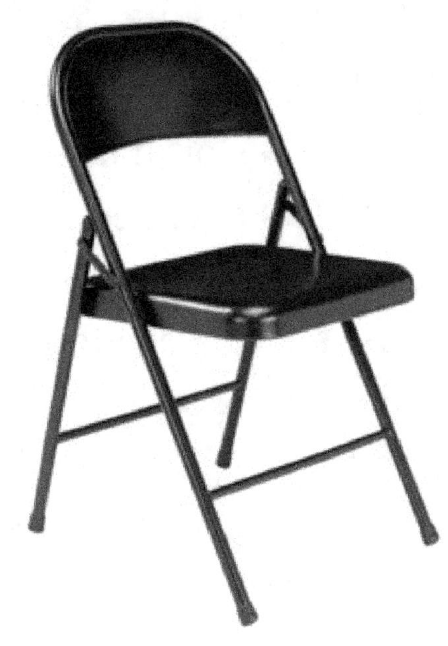

Picture of a sturdy chair for yoga

Safety Precautions and Guidelines

Safety is crucial in any workout practice, including chair yoga. Here are some safety considerations and tips to bear in mind while doing chair yoga.

Listen to your body: Pay attention to how your body feels throughout practice, and respect your limitations. If something doesn't feel right or causes discomfort, stop immediately and adjust the position to your requirements.

Move Mindfully: Move through each position slowly and thoughtfully, focusing on mindfulness and awareness. Avoid making quick or jerky movements that may strain your muscles or joints.

Stay Hydrated: Drink lots of water before, during, and after your practice to avoid dehydration.

Use Props for Support: Don't be afraid to use props like cushions, blankets, or yoga blocks to help support your body and improve your practice. These props can help you stay in perfect alignment and avoid injury.

Consult Your Healthcare Physician: Before beginning a chair yoga practice, discuss any current health issues or concerns with your healthcare physician. They can offer unique advice and recommendations based on your specific requirements and constraints.

Practice regularly: Consistency is essential for receiving the advantages of chair yoga. Aim to practice consistently, even if it's only for a few minutes each day. Your flexibility, strength, and overall well-being will increase with time.

By adhering to these safety measures and instructions, you may have a safe and pleasurable chair yoga practice that benefits your health and wellness.

Chapter 2: Gentle Chair Yoga Poses for Seniors of All Levels

Chair yoga is an excellent kind of yoga that may be enjoyed and benefited by individuals of all ages and abilities. The beauty of chair yoga is that it requires simply a chair and a small amount of space. There are many chair yoga postures to try, and in this chapter, we'll look at some of the most popular. We'll also look at the advantages of each position and how to do them safely. With a little practice, you'll be able to identify the chair yoga postures that are most effective for you and your specific requirements and skills.

This chapter delves further into the advantages and practices of chair yoga, including how these poses may help you improve your flexibility, strength, and balance from the convenience of your chair. Whether you're new to yoga or a seasoned practitioner, this chapter will walk you through a series of chair yoga positions that you can simply include in your everyday practice.

As we explore these chair yoga positions, remember to move carefully and listen to your body. Each posture has its own set of advantages, and it's crucial to respect your body's limitations while still pushing yourself to grow and improve. Regular practice can not only enhance your physical health but also give you a better feeling of calm and well-being.

So, take a chair, locate a comfy spot, and let's start exploring chair yoga positions together.

Introduction to Gentle Chair Yoga Poses

Do you remember Maria, my Aunt? Okay, I think you do. And if you don't, I recommend that you reread the book's introduction. You, like Maria, a reluctant beginner to yoga who originally found the practice intimidating and unfamiliar since it needs a shift in thinking and approach, may face hurdles when you embark on your chair yoga journey. It's normal to feel hesitant or scared, especially if you're used to more traditional types of exercise. However, I encourage you to approach this chapter with an open heart and mind, eager to experience yoga's transformational potential. Remember that yoga is more than simply physical poses; it's a whole practice that benefits the body, mind, and soul. I ask you to let go of any preconceived assumptions or self-doubt and instead nurture an attitude of inquiry, boldness, and self-care.

1. Seated Mountain Pose (Tadasana).

i. Begin by sitting up straight in your chair, feet flat on the floor, hands resting on your thighs

ii. Activate your core muscles and stretch your spine, seeing yourself rising taller with each breath and your hands now slowly rising above your head.

iii. Hold this posture for many breaths with your shoulders relaxed and your eyes ahead, feeling anchored and grounded like a mountain.

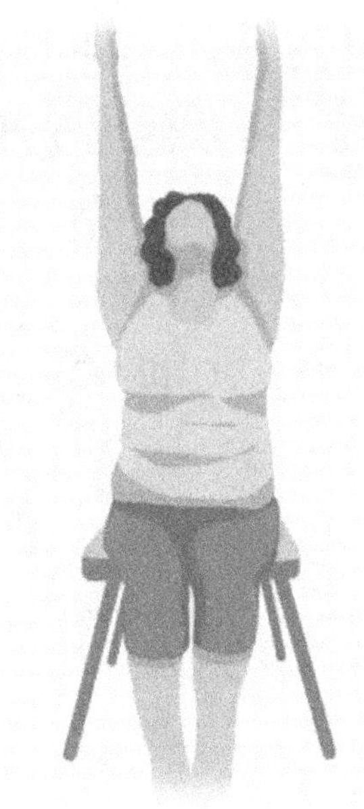

Seated mountain pose

Benefits:

- It improves posture and alignment.
- Strengthens core muscles.
- Encourages a sense of anchoring and solidity.
- Reduces strain in the shoulders and upper back.

2. Seated Cat-Cow Stretch.

i. Begin by sitting up straight in your chair, feet flat on the floor, hands resting on your thighs.

ii. Inhale while arching your back and lifting your chest to the ceiling, bringing your shoulder blades together.

iii. Exhale as you circle your back, tuck your chin to your chest, and bring your belly button towards your spine.

iv. Repeat this flowing motion with your breath, gradually extending and mobilizing your spine.

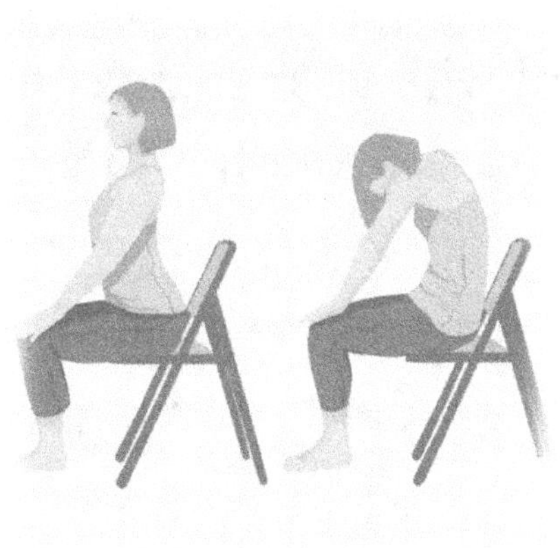

Seated Cat-Cow Stretch.

Benefits:
- Increases spinal flexibility and mobility.
- Reduces stress in the back, neck, and shoulders.
- It stimulates the digestive functions.
- Boosts circulation and energy levels throughout the body.

3. Seated Forward Fold (Paschimottanasana).

i.   Sit up straight in your chair, feet flat on the floor, hands resting on your thighs.

ii. Inhale to extend your spine, then exhale as you bend forward from your hips, reaching your hands for your feet or the floor.

iii. Fold forward with your spine extended and chest elevated, allowing your head to relax towards your knees.

iv. Hold this pose for a few breaths until you feel a slight stretch in your hamstrings and lower back.

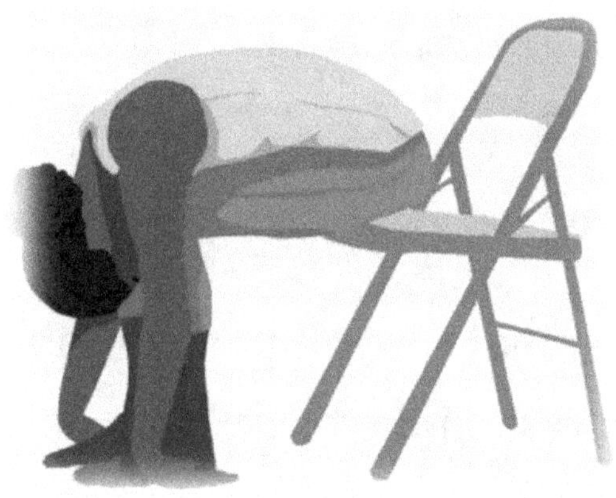

Seated Forward Fold

Benefits:
- Stretch the hamstrings and calves.
- Reduces tightness in the lower back.
- Relaxes the mind and relieves tension.
- It stimulates the gastrointestinal organs and helps digestion.

4. Seated Twist (Ardha Matsyendrasana).

i. Sit up straight in your chair, feet flat on the floor, hands resting on your thighs.

ii. Inhale as you stretch your spine, then exhale as you rotate your body to the right, with your left hand on the outside of your right leg and your right hand on the chair's back.

iii. With each exhale, deepen the twist while keeping your spine long and shoulders relaxed.

iv. Hold this posture for a few breaths before repeating on the opposing side.

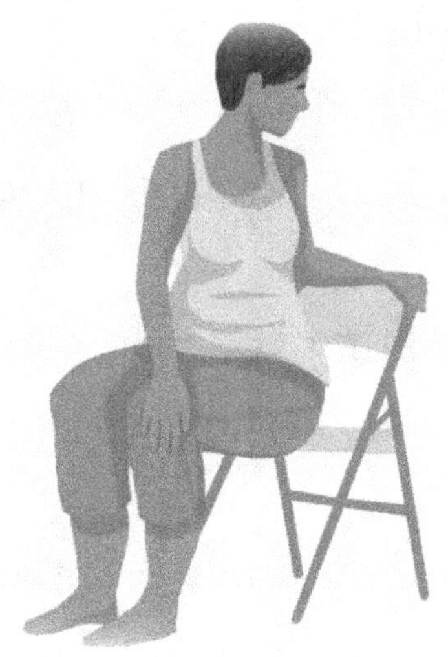

Seated Twist

Benefits:

- Increases spinal mobility and flexibility.

- Massages the abdominal organs to improve digestion.
- Reduces stress in the back, shoulders, and neck.
- Detoxifies the body and improves general health.

5. Seated Warrior Pose (Virabhadrasana).

i. Sit up straight in your chair, feet flat on the floor, hands resting on your thighs.

ii. Extend your right leg to the side, keeping your foot flat on the ground.

iii. Inhale as you raise your arms upwards and reach for the ceiling.

iv. Exhale while leaning your torso towards your right leg, experiencing a stretch on the left side of your body.

v. Hold this posture for a few breaths before repeating on the opposing side.

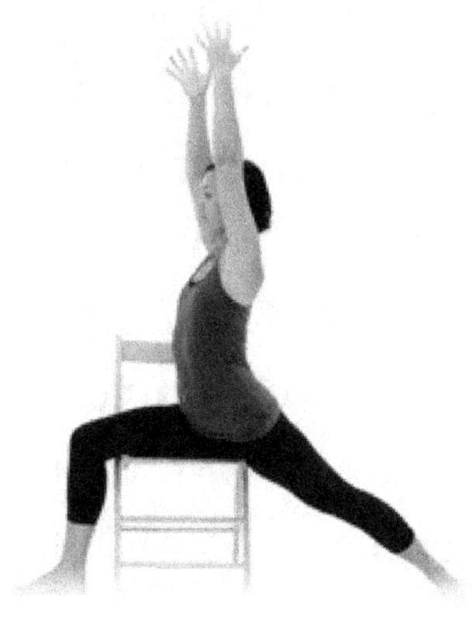

Seated Warrior Pose

Benefits:

- Strengthens the legs, hips, and core muscles.
- It promotes balance and stability.
- Opens the chest and shoulders, which improves posture.
- Promotes mental clarity and concentration.

6. Seated tree pose (Vrksasana).

i. Sit up straight in your chair, feet flat on the floor, hands resting on your thighs.

ii.   Position your right foot on your left inner thigh, either above or below the knee.

iii. Inhale as you raise your arms upwards and reach for the ceiling.

iv.   Exhale as you place your right foot on your left thigh and stretch your spine.

v.   Hold this posture for a few breaths before repeating on the opposing side.

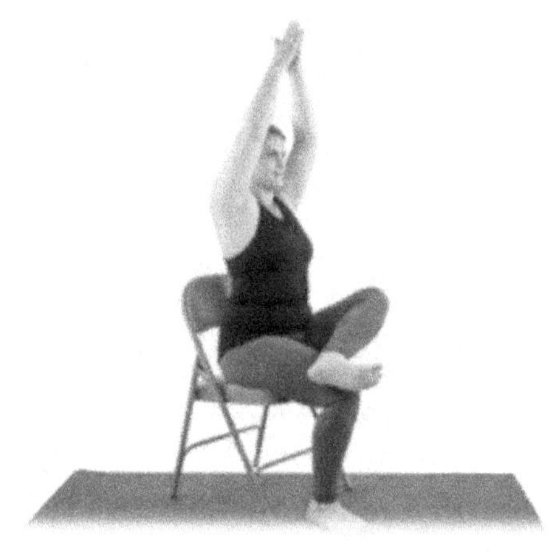

Seated tree pose

Benefits:

- It promotes balance and stability.
- Increases leg and core muscular strength.
- Opens and extends the hips and inner thighs.
- Increases serenity and mental clarity.

Explore these chair yoga postures at your speed, and don't be afraid to experiment with variations and changes to meet your specific requirements. With consistent practice, you'll notice better flexibility, strength, and balance, as well as a heightened sense of calm and well-being.

Sitting stretches and breathing exercises

Seniors over the age of 60 might benefit greatly from sitting stretches and breathing exercises. These mild exercises help boost flexibility, circulation, and strength without putting undue strain on the body. They may be done anywhere, at any time, and require no specific equipment or gym membership. They're also an excellent method to maintain your fitness, health, and happiness as you become older.

Seated stretches are great for gradually lengthening and loosening tight muscles, especially in the neck, shoulders, back, and hips. Gentle motions and stretches can help relieve stiffness, improve flexibility, and increase general mobility. Furthermore, breathing exercises are an effective strategy for lowering stress and anxiety, improving mental clarity, and increasing sensations of relaxation and well-being.

I invite you to study and practice these sitting stretches and breathing exercises while keeping an open mind and a kind heart. With regular practice, your flexibility, circulation, and strength will improve over time. Listen to your body, acknowledge its limitations, and practice with mindfulness and awareness. Remember that the actual core of yoga is not seeking perfection, but rather building a deeper connection with oneself and finding joy in the now.

So, locate a peaceful and comfortable area, sit in your favorite chair, and let's start with sitting stretches and breathing exercises. May each soft movement and focused breath bring you a refreshed sense of well-being, balance, and vigor.

Seated stretches:

Neck Stretch:

i. Sit tall on your chair, feet flat on the floor.

ii. Inhale and extend your spine.

iii. Exhale and slowly lower your right ear to your right shoulder.

iv. Remain in the stretch for 15-30 seconds, inhaling deeply.

v. Inhale to return to the center, then repeat on the opposite side.

vi. Repeat 2-3 times per side.

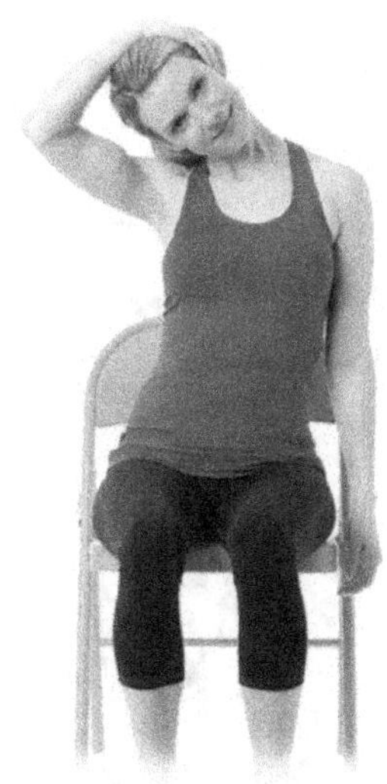

Neck stretches

Benefits:

- Reduces stress and stiffness in the neck and shoulders.

- It improves neck range of motion.

- Reduces headaches and neck discomfort.

- It promotes relaxation and decreases tension.

Shoulder Roll:

   i.   Sit tall, arms at your sides.

  ii.   Inhale and raise your shoulders to your ears.

 iii.   Exhale, then roll your shoulders back and down in a circular manner.

 iv.   Repeat for 10-15 times.

  v.   Reverse the direction of the shoulder roll for an additional 10-15 repetitions.

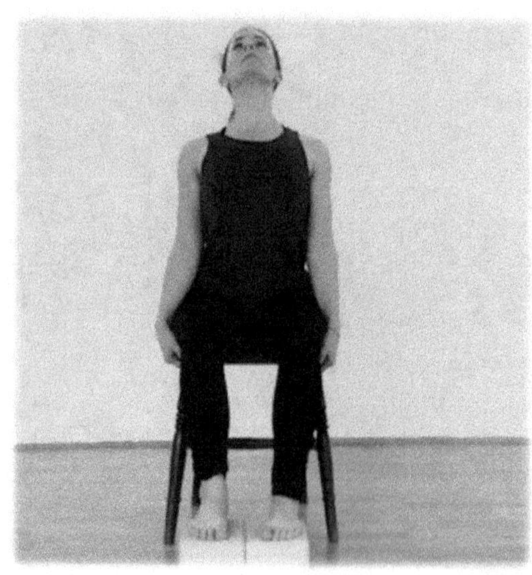

Shoulder roll

Benefits:

- Reduces strain in the shoulders and upper back.
- Increases circulation to the shoulder region.
- Raises awareness of posture and body alignment.
- Reduces shoulder stiffness and pain.

Side Stretch:

i. Sit tall, feet flat on the floor, arms at your sides.

ii. Inhale and extend your spine.

iii. Exhale and stretch your right arm up and across to the left side, bending slightly to the left.

iv. Remain in the stretch for 15-30 seconds, inhaling deeply.

v. Inhale to return to the center, then repeat on the opposite side.

vi. Repeat 2-3 times per side.

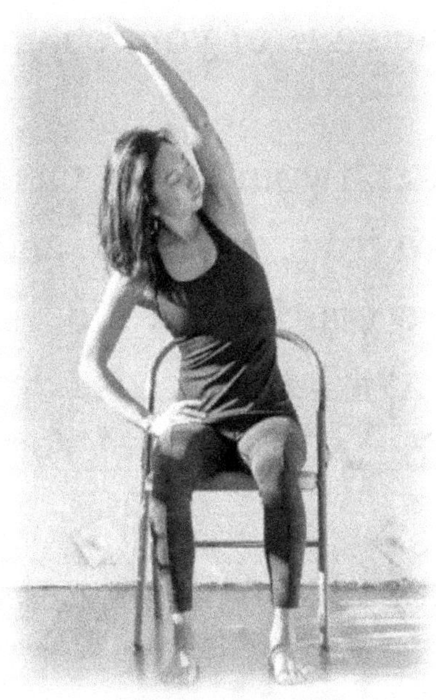

Side stretch

Benefits:

- Stretch the sides of the body, especially the intercostal muscles.
- Increases spinal and ribcage flexibility.
- Expands lung capacity and encourages deeper breathing.
- Reduces strain in the waist and lower back.

Seated Forward Bend:

i. Sit tall on the edge of your chair, feet flat on the floor.

ii. Inhale to extend your spine, then exhale as you bend forward from your hips and stretch your hands toward your feet or the floor.

iii. Let your head relax towards your knees, then hold the stretch for 15-30 seconds while inhaling deeply.

iv. Inhale to get back to a sitting position.

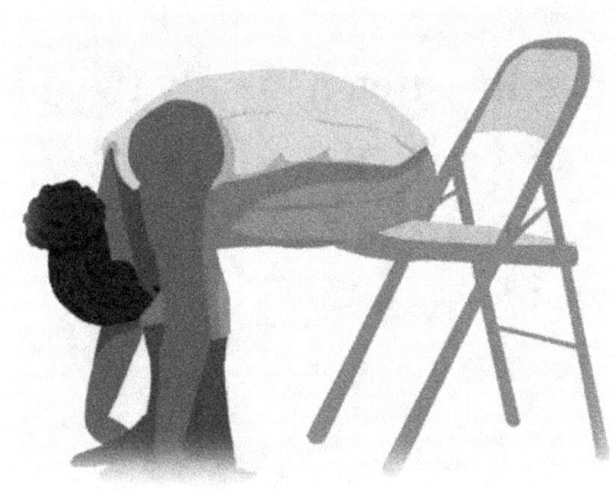

Seated Forward Bend

Benefits:

- It stretches the hamstrings and lower back muscles.
- Reduces spinal tension and tightness.
- Calms the mind and relieves tension and anxiety.
- Boosts digestion and improves bowel function.

Seated Spinal Twist:

i. Sit tall on your chair, feet flat on the floor.

ii. Inhale to stretch your spine, then exhale and rotate your body to the right, with your left hand on the outside of your right leg and your right hand on the back of the chair.

iii. To deepen the stretch, gently twist and hold for 15-30 seconds while inhaling deeply.

iv. Inhale to return to the center, then repeat on the opposite side.

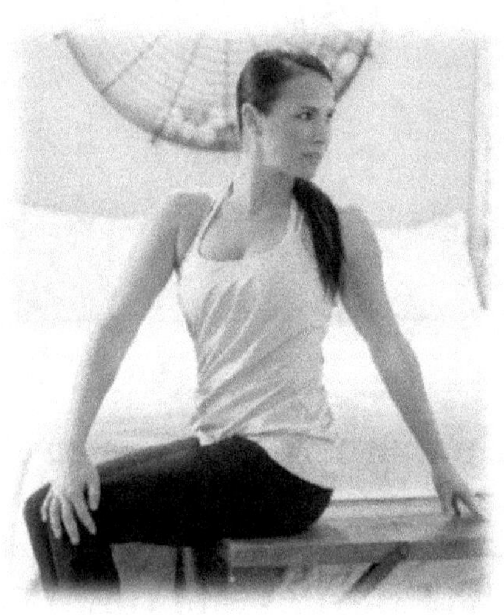

Seated Spinal Twist

Benefits:

- It improves spinal mobility and flexibility.
- Reduces stress in the spine, hips, and lower back.
- It stimulates the digestive system and assists in cleansing.
- Boosts circulation in the abdomen region.

Seated Hip Opener:

  i.   Sit tall on your chair, feet flat on the floor.
 ii.   Cross your right ankle over your left knee and flex your right foot.
iii.   Inhale to lengthen your spine, then exhale while softly pressing down on your right knee, experiencing a stretch in your right hip and outer thigh.
iv.   Hold the stretch for 15-30 seconds while breathing deeply, then repeat on the opposite side.

Benefits:

- It stretches the hip flexors, outer hips, and glutes.
- It enhances hip mobility and range of motion.
- Reduces stress and stiffness in the hips and lower back.
- It promotes relaxation and reduces tension and anxiety.

Breathing exercises:

Deep belly breathing (sometimes called diaphragmatic breathing):

-Sit comfortably, feet flat on the floor, hands resting on your thighs.

-Close your eyes and take a deep breath in through your nose, feeling your tummy expand as you inhale.
-Slowly exhale via your lips, moving your belly button towards your spine.
-Continue to breathe deeply, concentrating on full your lungs with each inhalation and completely emptying them with each exhalation.
-Start with 3-5 minutes of practice and progressively increase the time as you gain confidence in the technique.

Benefits:

-Increases relaxation and decreases tension and anxiety.
-Increases lung function and respiratory efficiency.
-Boosts oxygenation in the blood and tissues.
-Helps control the autonomic nervous system and promotes serenity.

Alternate nostril breathing (Nadi Shodhana):
-Sit comfortably, keeping your spine tall and your shoulders relaxed.
-Place your left hand on your left knee, palm facing up.

i. Put your right hand to your face, index and middle fingers on your forehead, between your eyebrows.
ii. Close your right nostril with your thumb and breathe deeply through your left nose.
iii. Close your left nostril with your ring finger, then gently exhale through your right.
iv. Inhale via your right nostril, then shut it with your thumb and breathe out through your left nose.
v. Repeat this alternate nostril breathing pattern for numerous rounds, concentrating on the flow of your breath and keeping a smooth, steady pace.

Breath (equal breathing):
i. Sit comfortably, with your spine upright and your hands resting on your thighs.
ii. To focus on yourself, close your eyes and take several deep breaths.
iii. Take a calm, steady inhale through your nostrils for four counts.
iv. Take a calm and steady exhale through your nostrils for four counts.
v. Repeat this rhythm of breathing and exhaling for numerous rounds, progressively increasing the count as you feel comfortable.

vi. Repeat this pattern for many rounds, focusing on the sensations of coldness on the inhale and warmth on the exhale.

vii. Maintain an identical duration for both inhale and exhale to keep your breathing smooth and steady.

Benefits:

- Calms the mind and relieves tension and anxiety.
- Increases attention, concentration, and mental clarity.
- Regulates the autonomic nerve system and promotes relaxation.
- Increases self-awareness and attention in the current moment.

Box breathing (or square breathing):

i. Sit comfortably, with your spine upright and your hands resting on your thighs.

ii. Inhale deeply and steadily through your nose for a count of four.

iii. Hold your breath at the peak of the inhale for four counts.

iv. Take a calm and steady exhale through your nostrils for four counts.

v. Hold your breath at the bottom of the exhale for four counts.

vi. Repeat this pattern multiple times, focusing on the rhythm of your breath and keeping equal counts for each phase.

Benefits:

- Creates a mood of peace and relaxation.
- It regulates the breath and balances the neurological system.
- Increases attention, concentration, and mental clarity.
- Assists with stress, anxiety, and overload.

Lions Breath (Simhasana Pranayama):

i. Sit comfortably, with your spine upright and your hands resting on your thighs.

ii. Inhale deeply through your nose to fill your lungs with air.

iii. Forcefully exhale through your mouth, thrust out your tongue, and roar like a lion.

iv. Repeat 2-3 times, letting yourself expel tension and stress with each breath.

Benefits:

- Eliminates tension and stagnation in the face and throat.
- It clears the sinuses and promotes the respiratory system.
- Energizes the body and stimulates the intellect.
- Creates a feeling of release and freedom.

Sitali Pranayama (Cool Breath):

i. Sit comfortably, with your spine upright and your hands resting on your thighs.

ii. If you can't roll your tongue into a tube, purse your lips instead.

iii. Inhale deeply through your mouth, bringing the breath in with your rolled tongue or pursed lips.

iv. Exhale gently and steadily via the nose.

Benefits:

- Reduces body temperature and inflammation.
- Calms the mind, reducing anger, frustration, and impatience.
- Reduces thirst and refreshes the lips and throat.
- Improves and calms the digestive system.

Regularly practice these sitting stretches and breathing exercises to improve your relaxation, flexibility, and general health. Remember to listen to your body and alter the workouts to meet your specific demands and comfort level. Enjoy your practice!

Mindful Movement Techniques for Seniors.

Mindful movement entails focusing attention on the present moment while moving with intention, awareness, and purpose. As we age, it is critical to maintain and improve our physical function to retain independence and quality of life. Mindful movement techniques provide a gentle yet effective way to attain these objectives, helping seniors to move more easily, gracefully, and confidently. Seniors who practice mindfulness while moving can create a stronger connection to their body, minimize the chance of injury, and improve lifespan and vitality. Throughout this part, we will look at several mindful movement practices that are appropriate for seniors of different levels and abilities. These techniques range from basic sitting stretches to dynamic standing motions, providing a comprehensive approach to maintaining and increasing physical health and function. Whether you want to gain flexibility, strengthen muscles, or improve your balance and coordination, you'll discover a variety of exercises and practices to meet your specific requirements and goals.

Seated Body Scan:

i. Sit comfortably in a chair, feet flat on the floor, hands resting on your thighs.

ii. To focus on yourself, close your eyes and take several deep breaths.

iii. Start with your feet and gradually increase your awareness of your body, noting any places of tension, pain, or relaxation.

iv. Take your time scanning your whole body, from your feet to your legs, hips, chest, arms, shoulders, neck, and head.

v. Notice any sensations without judgment or opposition, allowing oneself to completely engage in the present moment.

Benefits:

- Increases bodily awareness and mindfulness.
- Identifies areas of tension or discomfort, allowing for more focused alleviation.

- Encourages relaxation and stress reduction.
- Improves mental clarity and concentration.

Mindful Walking:

i. Look for a peaceful and safe area where you may stroll easily, such as a corridor or garden.

ii. Start by standing tall, feet hip-width apart, and arms relaxed at your sides.

iii. Take a few deep breaths to center yourself, paying attention to the feelings in your body.

iv. Begin walking slowly and deliberately, paying attention to every step you take.

v. Take note of the sensation of your feet on the ground, the movement of your legs and arms, and the rhythm of your breathing.

vi. If your thoughts begin to stray, gently return your focus to the current moment and the act of walking.

Benefits:

- Enhances balance and coordination.
- Strengthens the leg muscles and promotes joint health.
- Improves cardiovascular health and circulation.

- Relieves tension and anxiety via rhythmic movement and breathing awareness.

Chair Yoga Flow:
i. Sit tall on a solid chair, feet flat on the floor, hands resting on your thighs.
ii. Start with a few deep breaths to ground yourself and reconnect with your body.
iii. Perform a sequence of easy yoga postures modified for the chair, including sitting cat-cow stretches, seated twists, and moderate forward folds.
iv. Coordinate your motions with your breath, inhaling to lengthen and exhaling to deepen the stretch.
v. Pay attention to how each action feels and how your breath connects to your body.
vi. Adjust the postures as required to meet your specific requirements and skills, and always heed your body's signals.

Benefits:
- improves flexibility and range of motion.
- Improves strength and muscular tone.

- Improves posture and alignment.
- Promotes relaxation and relieves muscular tension.

Joint mobilization exercises:

i. Sit comfortably in a chair, feet flat on the floor, hands on your lap.

ii. Start by gently moving each joint in your body through its complete range of motion, beginning with your fingers and toes and then progressing to your wrists, ankles, elbows, shoulders, hips, and neck.

iii. Move gently and deliberately, paying attention to any areas of stiffness or discomfort.

iv. Let your breath lead the motions, inhaling as you extend and exhaling as you release.

v. Repeat each action numerous times, letting your muscles relax and soften with each one.

Benefits:

- Improves joint flexibility and mobility.
- Reduces the stiffness and pain caused by arthritis or aging.
- Promotes joint health and lifespan.

- Improves overall physical performance and range of motion.

Breath Awareness Meditation:
i. Sit comfortably in a chair, feet flat on the floor, hands resting on your thighs.
ii. To focus on yourself, close your eyes and take several deep breaths.
iii. Pay attention to your breath, feeling the sensation of air going in and out of your body.
iv. Observe the natural rhythm of your breath without attempting to alter it in any way.
v. If your mind wanders, gently return your focus to your breath, which serves as an anchor to the present moment.
vi. Sit and breathe attentively for a few minutes, allowing yourself to feel quiet and relaxed.
vii. Incorporate these mindful movement practices into your daily routine to improve physical health, emotional well-being, and energy.

Remember to practice with patience, curiosity, and self-compassion, while respecting your body's own needs and talents. Enjoy your journey via mindful exercise!

Benefits:
- Relaxes the neurological system and relieves tension.
- Improves mental clarity and concentration.
- Develops a sense of inner calm and well-being.
- Enhances respiratory function and lung capacity.

Seated Spinal Twist:
i.   Sit upright on a chair, feet flat on the floor and hands resting on your thighs.
ii. Inhale to stretch your spine, then exhale and rotate your body to the right, with your left hand on the outside of your right leg and your right hand on the back of the chair.
iii. Remain in the twist for a few breaths, experiencing the mild stretch over your spine and torso.
iv. Inhale to return to the center, then repeat on the opposite side.

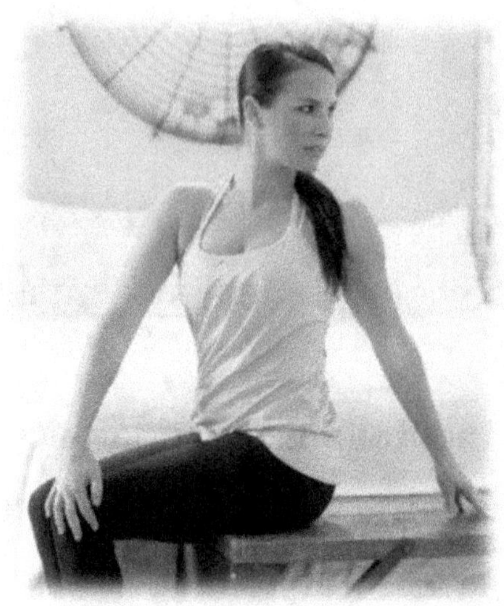

Seated Spinal Twist

Benefits:

- Improves spinal mobility and flexibility.
- Promotes digestion and assists in cleansing.
- Reduces stress and stiffness in the back and shoulders.
- Enhances posture and spinal alignment.

Seated Leg Extensions:

i. Sit upright on a chair, feet flat on the floor and hands resting on your thighs.

ii. Inhale to lengthen your spine, then exhale and stretch your right leg straight out in front of you, flexing your foot.

iii. Remain in place for a few breaths, experiencing the stretch in your hamstring and calf.

iv. Inhale to bend your knee and return to the beginning position, then repeat on the opposite side.

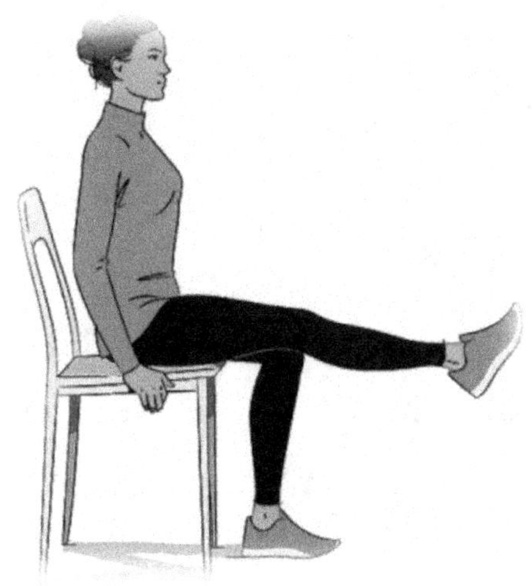

Seated Leg Extensions

Benefits:

- It strengthens the quadriceps and calf muscles.
- Improves circulation in the lower extremities.
- Improves the flexibility and range of motion in the legs.
- Promotes joint health and lowers the chance of injury.

Chair Yoga Sun Salutation:

   i.   Sit upright on a chair, feet flat on the floor and hands resting on your thighs.

  ii.   Inhale as you sweep your arms upwards, reaching for the heavens.

 iii.   Exhale as you tilt forward from your hips, lowering your hands to the floor or your shins.

 iv.   Inhale and raise halfway, stretching your spine and reaching your chest forward.

  v.   Exhale to fold forward again, relieving tension in your neck and shoulders.

 vi.   Inhale, sweep your arms overhead and return to a sitting position.

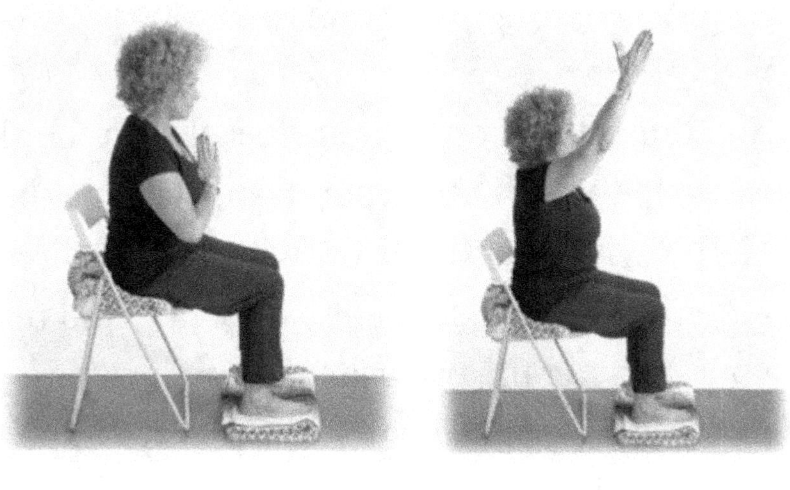

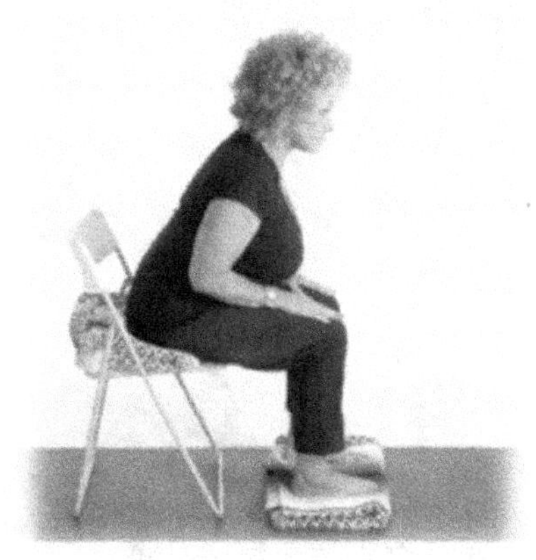

Chair Yoga Sun Salutation

Benefits:

- Improves general flexibility and mobility.
- Enhances circulation and blood flow throughout the body.
- Energizes the body and elevates the mood.
- Develops a sense of appreciation and attentiveness.

Ankle circles:

  i. Sit comfortably on a chair, feet flat on the floor.

  ii. Lift one foot off the ground and start making circles with your ankle, moving in one direction.

  iii. After a few circles, change direction and move your ankle in the opposite direction.

  iv. Repeat the exercise with the opposite foot, circling the ankle in both directions.

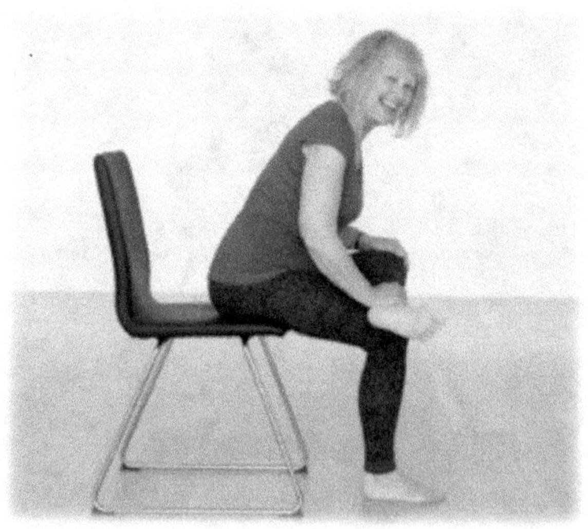

Ankle circles

Benefits:

- Increases ankle flexibility and mobility.
- Strengthens the muscles around the ankle joint.
- Lowers the risk of ankle injury and falls.

- Improves proprioception and balance.

Seated mountain pose:
  i.   Sit upright on a chair, feet flat on the floor and hands resting on your thighs.
  ii. Inhale to extend your spine and raise the top of your head to the heavens.
  iii. Push down through your sit bones and envision roots emerging from your tailbone into the ground underneath you.
  iv. Remain in this posture for a few breaths, feeling grounded and focused in your body.

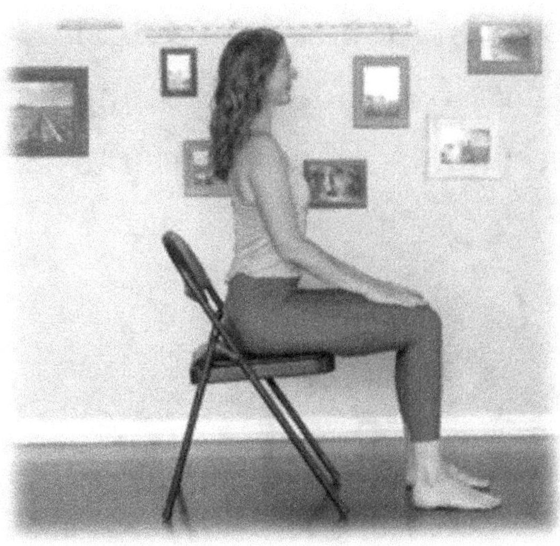

Seated mountain pose

Benefits:

- Promotes proper posture and spinal alignment.
- Strengthens core muscles and helps to stabilize the spine.
- Improves attention and mental focus.
- Promotes a sense of grounding and solidity.

Remember to practice with patience, curiosity, and self-compassion, while respecting your body's own needs and talents. Enjoy your journey via mindful exercise!

Chapter 3: Chair Yoga for Balance and Stability

When I was much younger, there was a man named Jack who lived a few blocks away. Jack was an adventurous man who spent most of his youth discovering nature's beauties. He was the one who climbed trees, rode his bike down winding paths, and danced in the rain with no worries in the world. Jack's enthusiasm for life and love of the outdoors was contagious, motivating everyone around him to experience the joys of movement and adventure. However, as Jack got older, the difficulties of life began to weigh on him. The previously carefree kid was confronted with the reality of maturing, including changes in his balance and stability. It appeared that the earth beneath his feet was shifting, threatening to deprive him of the freedom and vigor he had always valued.

Despite the failures, Jack maintained his adventurous attitude. He remembered the sense of liberation and exhilaration that came from being in tune with his body and the world around him. This recollection inspired his ambition to restore balance and stability, much like the trees he had adored as a child.

So, with a sense of nostalgia and a desire for the simplicity of childhood, Jack came to the garden of his recollections, seeking peace and inspiration in the natural beauty. As he sat beneath the canopy of trees, feeling the pleasant air on his face and the dirt beneath his feet, he recognized that the key to recovering his equilibrium was not battling against the currents of time, but rather submitting to his body's wisdom and the rhythm of life itself.

So, with newfound purpose and a heart full of optimism, Jack set out on a new journey—one that would take him to the practice of chair yoga. For in the smooth flow of movement and the thoughtful embrace of breath, he found a way back to himself, illuminated by nature's ageless wisdom and the unbounded spirit of his youthful fantasies.

Whether you're recuperating from an accident, managing a chronic disease, or simply wanting to keep your balance as you get older, chair yoga provides useful skills and approaches. By exercising consistently and mindfully, you may improve your ability to move with elegance, poise, and confidence in all parts of your life.

In this section of the book, we'll look at the significance of balance and stability for seniors, the underlying causes of balance problems, and practical chair yoga techniques for increasing balance. We'll also discuss typical balancing issues and obstacles, such as fear of falling and loss of mobility, and provide advice on how to overcome them with compassion and determination.

Importance of Balance and Stability in Aging

As we progress through life's phases, keeping balance and stability becomes increasingly important, particularly as we age. The capacity to stay firm on our feet, manage uneven terrain, and respond quickly to unforeseen difficulties is critical for maintaining independence, reducing falls, and improving overall quality of life.

Preventing Falls and Injury

Falls are the primary cause of injury and disability among the elderly, frequently resulting in fractures, brain injuries, and other significant effects. Seniors can retain their mobility and autonomy by increasing their balance and stability, lowering their risk of falling, and reducing the possibility of harm.

Supporting Functional Independence:
Walking, rising from a chair, and reaching for items above the head all need balance and stability. By improving these fundamental abilities, seniors may continue to do daily chores with confidence and ease, retaining their functional independence and quality of life.

Improving Mobility and Confidence:
Changes in muscular strength, joint flexibility, and sensory perception can all influence our capacity to move quickly and confidently as we age. Seniors who focus on balance and stability training can enhance their mobility, coordination, and proprioception, allowing them to traverse their environment with more confidence and elegance.

Promoting Cognitive Function:
According to research, there is a considerable correlation between physical balance and cognitive

performance. Activities that require balance and coordination can activate neuronal pathways in the brain, promoting cognitive health and lowering the risk of cognitive decline caused by aging.

Improving quality of life:

Maintaining balance and stability is critical for sustaining our general health and quality of life as we age. By engaging in proactive efforts to improve balance, seniors can experience more flexibility, autonomy, and involvement in meaningful activities, encouraging a sense of vitality and purpose in their golden years.

Preventing Fractures and Hospitalization:

Falls caused by poor balance can result in fractures, necessitating hospitalization and extended healing times. Seniors who prioritize balance and stability training can greatly reduce their risk of falling, decreasing the incidence of fractures and hospital visits.

Enhancing Postural Alignment:

Good balance and stability help to achieve good postural alignment, which reduces pressure on the spine and joints. Improved posture can reduce the discomfort and suffering caused by improper alignment, enabling greater spinal health and general comfort.

Supporting activities of daily living (ADLs):
Dressing, bathing, and cooking are all basic everyday tasks that demand a certain level of balance and stability. Seniors who enhance these abilities via focused exercises can execute ADLs more quickly and comfortably, preserving their independence and self-sufficiency.

Boosting Energy and Vitality:
Maintaining balance and stability promotes effective movement patterns while conserving energy during regular tasks. Seniors who emphasize balance training frequently report feeling more energetic and vibrant, allowing them to participate in a broader range of activities and have a greater quality of life.

Reducing fear of falling:
Fear of falling is a prevalent issue among seniors, which can result in decreased mobility and social isolation. Seniors who improve their balance and stability might gain confidence in their ability to walk safely and confidently, lowering their fear of falling and increasing their involvement in everyday life.

Improving Sleep Quality:

Regular exercise, particularly balance and stability training, has been found to improve the quality of sleep in older persons. Seniors who incorporate chair yoga and other balance-enhancing activities into their daily routine may have improved sleep patterns and general well-being.

Fostering Social Connections:

Participating in group balance and stability programs, such as chair yoga, allows for social connection and community participation. Connecting with peers who have similar health objectives might help you feel more at ease and supported as you age.

Recognizing the various advantages of balance and stability training allows seniors to make educated decisions about their physical and mental well-being as they age. Through constant practice and devotion, people may grow resilience, confidence, and vigor to face the difficulties and possibilities of aging with grace and resilience.

Chair Yoga Poses for Improving Balance and Core Strength

In this part, we'll look at a range of chair yoga postures designed specifically to improve balance and core strength. While you may have seen some of these tactics before in this book, it's vital to recognize that the repetition has a purpose. The goal of this book is not to overload you with many positions but to present you with relevant and practical approaches that are suited to your specific requirements. Revisiting classic poses from various perspectives enables you to get better knowledge and enhance your practice, resulting in more benefits to your entire health and well-being.

Chair Cat-Cow Pose (Marjarya-Bitilasana Variation):

i. Begin by sitting up straight in your chair, feet flat on the floor, and hands resting on your thighs.
ii. As you inhale, arch your back and raise your chest to the heavens, bringing your shoulder blades together.

iii. Exhale while rounding your back, tucking your chin to your chest, and pulling your navel towards your spine.

iv. Flow fluidly between these two motions, matching your breath to the motion of your spine.

v. Engage your core muscles while maintaining pelvic and hip stability.

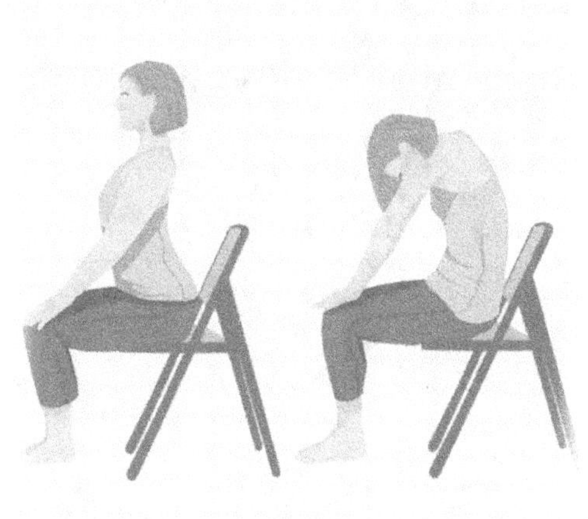

Chair Warrior I pose (Virabhadrasana I variation):

i. Sit at the front edge of your chair, feet hip-width apart and firmly planted on the floor.

ii.   Extend one leg straight behind you, toes pointing forward, heel elevated.

iii. Bend your front knee so it is squarely over your ankle, and use your core muscles to stabilize your spine.

iv.   Lift your arms above, reaching for the heavens with your fingers and dragging your shoulder blades down your spine.

v.   Hold the posture for a few breaths, feeling the strength and stability develop in your legs and core.

vi.   Repeat on the other side.

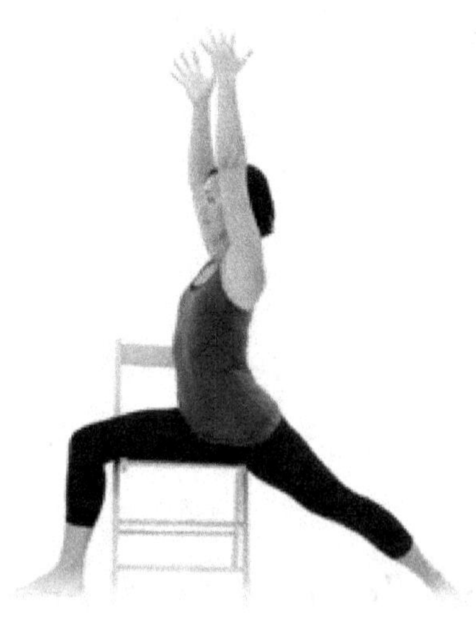

Chair Warrior I pose

Chair Eagle Pose (Garudasana variation):

i. Begin by sitting tall in your chair, feet flat on the floor, arms at your side.

ii. Cross one thigh over the other, then bring your knees together and stack them on top of each other.

iii. Wrap the upper foot around the calf of the standing leg, if feasible, or just push the foot against the shin for support.

iv. Extend your arms out to the sides at shoulder height, then cross them in front of your body, elbows bent and palms together.

v. Engage your core muscles to stay balanced and deepen the stretch over your shoulders and upper back.

vi. Hold the position for several breaths before releasing and repeating on the opposing side.

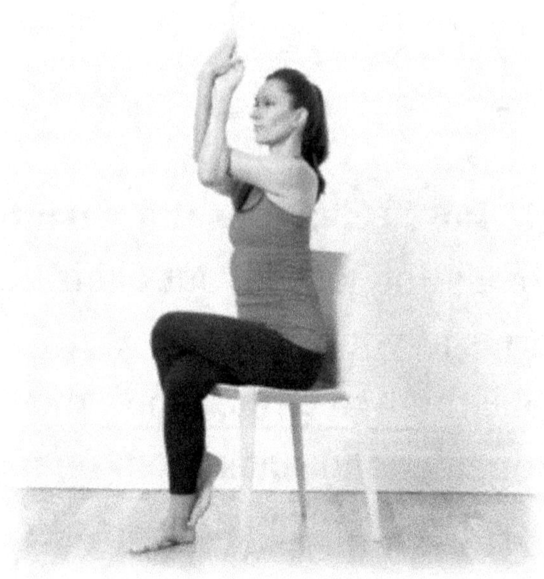

Chair Eagle Pose

Chair Boat Pose (Navasana variation):

i.   Sit at the front edge of your chair, feet flat on the floor, knees bent.

ii. Hold onto the chair's sides for support while leaning back slightly, raising your feet off the floor, and balancing on your sit bones.

iii. Maintain your balance by extending your arms forward at shoulder height, parallel to the floor, and using your core muscles.

iv. If you are comfortable, straighten your legs while maintaining them together and elevate at a 45-degree angle from the ground.

v. Hold the stance for several breaths, noticing the engagement of your core muscles and the sensation of buoyancy in your body.

vi. To release, gently lower your feet to the floor and sit back down.

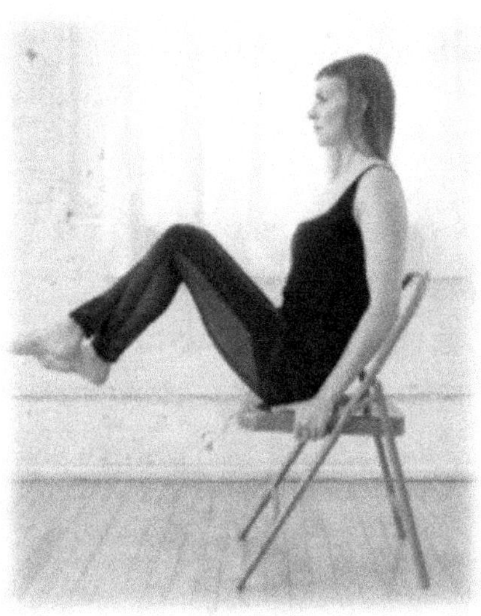

Chair Boat Pose

Chair Tree Pose (Vrksasana variation):

i. Begin by sitting tall in your chair, feet flat on the floor, hands resting on your thighs.

ii. Lift one foot off the floor and press the sole on the inner calf or thigh of your standing leg.

iii. To maintain balance, press your foot firmly into your leg and activate your core muscles.

iv. Bring your hands together at your heart's center, or stretch your arms upward for an extra challenge.

v. Hold the posture for a few breaths, feeling anchored and secure in your standing leg with a tall spine.

vi. Repeat on the other side.

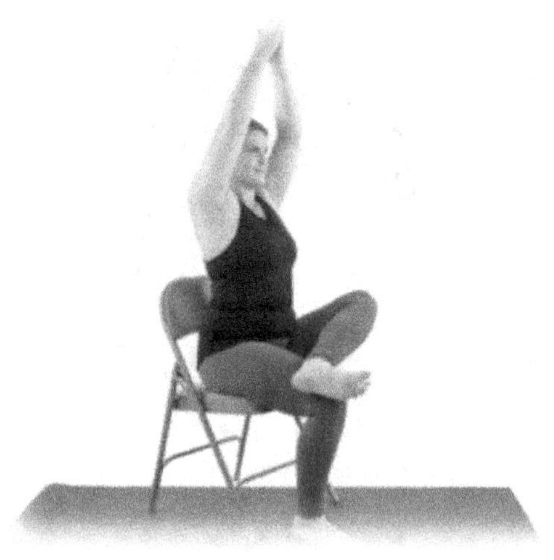

Chair Tree Pose

Chair Extended Side Angle Pose (a variation of Utthita Parsvakonasana):

i. Begin by sitting tall in your chair, feet flat on the floor, hands resting on your thighs.

ii. Extend one arm upwards, reaching for the opposite side of the room while keeping your other hand firmly on the chair.

iii. Engage your core muscles to stay stable and stretch your side body.

iv. If comfortable, look upward toward your outstretched hand, or keep your eyes ahead for increased stability.

v. Hold the position for a few breaths before switching sides to balance the stretch.

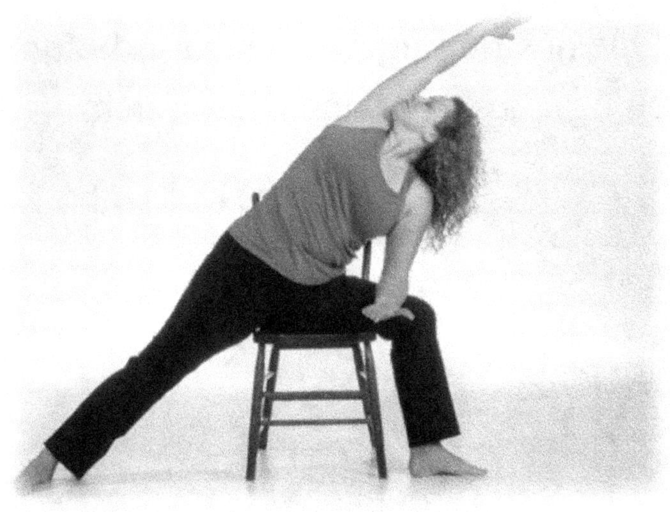

Chair Extended Side Angle Pose

Chair Warrior II Position (Virabhadrasana II Variation):

i. Sit at the front edge of your chair, feet hip-width apart and firmly planted on the floor.

ii. Extend one leg straight behind you, toes pointing forward, heel elevated.

iii. Bend your front knee, ensuring it is exactly over your ankle, and move your body to the side.

iv. Extend your arms to the sides, shoulder height, and reach through your fingertips.

v. Engage your core muscles to maintain your spine and extend the stretch into your inner thigh and hip.

vi. Hold the position for a few breaths before switching sides to balance the stretch.

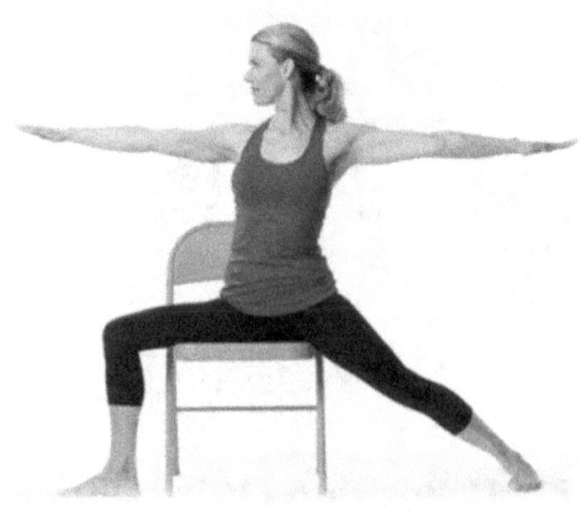

Chair Warrior II Position

Chairside Plank Pose (Vasisthasana Variation):

i. Begin by sitting sideways on your chair, one hand resting on the seat and the other stretched aloft.

ii. Lift your hips off the chair and form a side plank posture, keeping your body in a straight line from head to heels.

iii. Engage your core muscles to stay stable and prevent sinking into your shoulder.

iv. Hold the position for a few breaths, feeling your core and side body becoming stronger and more stable.

v. Repeat on the opposite side to even out the strain and strengthen both sides of your body.

Chair Boat Twist Pose (Paripurna Navasana variation):

i. Sit at the front edge of your chair, feet flat on the floor, knees bent.

ii. Lean back slightly, raise your feet off the ground, and balance on your sit bones.

iii. Extend your arms forward to shoulder height and parallel to the floor.

iv. Twist your body to one side and bring one elbow to the outside of the opposing knee.

v. Engage your core muscles to keep your balance and deepen the twist in your spine.

vi. Hold the position for a few breaths before returning to the center and repeating on the opposing side.

Chair High Lunge Pose (Anjaneyasana variation):

i. Sit at the front edge of your chair, feet hip-width apart and firmly planted on the floor.

ii. Extend one leg straight behind you, toes pointing forward, heel elevated.

iii. Bend your front knee, ensuring it is exactly over your ankle, and raise your arms overhead.

iv. Engage your core muscles to maintain your spine and increase the stretch in your hip flexors and quads.

v. Hold the posture for a few breaths, feeling the strength and stability develop in your legs and core.

vi. Repeat on the opposite side to even out the strain and strengthen both sides of your body.

vii.   Adding these chair yoga postures to your daily
       practice will help seniors improve their balance,
       stability, and core strength over time. As you
       experiment with each posture, remember to move
       thoughtfully, breathe deeply, and pay attention to
       your body's instructions.

       With patience, tenacity, and a sense of wonder,
       you may create increased resilience, energy, and
       well-being in your golden years.

Benefits of Chair Yoga for Improving Balance and Core Strength:

Enhanced stability and posture alignment:
Regular chair yoga postures that focus on balance and
core strength can assist improve stability and
alignment. Seniors can improve their posture and
lower their risk of falling by strengthening the muscles
that support their spine and pelvis.

Increased Muscle Strength:

Chair yoga positions work a multitude of muscles, including the core, legs, and arms. Over time, this can lead to greater muscular strength, which is necessary for completing daily tasks comfortably and lowering the chance of injury.

Improved balance and coordination:

Balancing postures in chair yoga need focus and coordination, which can assist improve balance over time. Enhanced proprioception—the body's knowledge of its location in space—can also help with balance and stability in daily living.

Improved Core Stability:

Core strength is necessary to support the spine and maintain appropriate posture. Chair yoga postures that work the core muscles—such as the abdominals, obliques, and lower back—can help develop these muscles, resulting in improved core stability and less back discomfort.

Increased Flexibility and Range of Motion:

Many chair yoga postures include mild stretching of the muscles and joints, which can aid with flexibility and range of motion. Increased flexibility can make daily chores simpler to complete while also reducing stiffness and discomfort caused by aging.

Stress Reduction and Relaxation:
Chair yoga classes frequently incorporate focused breathing and relaxation methods, which may help decrease stress and create a sense of peace and well-being. The emphasis on breath awareness can also help elders develop more mindfulness and resilience in the face of life's obstacles.

Improved circulation and energy flow:
Certain chair yoga positions can assist in increasing blood circulation and energy flow throughout the body. This can lead to improved general health and vigor, as well as a more positive feeling of well-being.

Increased Mental Clarity and Focus:
Chair yoga positions need attention and mental focus, which can aid in cognitive function and clarity. Seniors may find that frequent practice helps them stay focused and alert throughout the day.

Promoting Relaxation and Better Sleep:
Chair yoga positions that emphasize relaxation and moderate stretching will help you sleep better and relax more. Regular practice may result in better sleep quality and fewer symptoms of insomnia for seniors.

Empowerment and sense of accomplishment:
As seniors continue through their chair yoga practice
and discover gains in their balance, strength, and
overall well-being, they may feel empowered and
accomplished. This can enhance self-confidence and
drive to keep practicing and trying new positions.

Progression Exercises for Improved Stability

These exercises in this section expand on the core
postures taught previously in the book, providing
variations and adaptations to help you improve your
stability and confidence in your practice. Remember to
move thoughtfully, listen to your body, and only go to
more challenging exercises when you're ready.

Seated Warrior III Variation:

i. Begin by sitting tall in your chair, feet flat on the
   floor, hands resting on your thighs.
ii. Extend one leg straight back behind you, with your
    toes pointed and heel elevated.

iii. Lean forward slightly, stretching your arms forward at shoulder level and raising your extended leg to hip level.

iv. Maintain your balance by engaging your core muscles and lengthening your extended leg and spine.

v. Hold the posture for a few breaths before releasing and repeating on the opposing side.

Benefits:

- This version tests balance and proprioception, resulting in increased stability and coordination.
- Actively engages and strengthens the muscles of the standing leg, including the quadriceps, hamstrings, and glutes.
- Engage the core to maintain stability, develop the abdominal muscles, and improve posture.

Seated Side Plank Variation:

i. Sit at the front edge of your chair, feet level on the floor and hands resting on the seat.

ii. Lift your hips off the chair and form a side plank posture, keeping your body in a straight line from head to heels.

iii. Extend your upper arm overhead, reaching for the heavens, and use your core muscles to stay stable.

iv. Hold the position for a few moments before lowering your hips to the chair and repeating on the other side.

Benefits:

- Focuses on the obliques and deep core muscles to improve core strength and stability.
- Strengthens the arms, shoulders, and wrists, improving upper body stability and mobility.
- Tests coordination and balance while increasing general body awareness.

Chair Half Moon Pose:

i. Sit at the front edge of your chair, feet flat on the floor and hands resting on your thighs.

ii. Extend one leg straight out to the side, with your toes pointed and heel raised.

iii. Lean to the opposite side, stretching one arm down to the floor and the other up toward the sky.

iv. Use your core muscles to stay balanced and stretch through your extended leg and side body.

v. Hold the position for a few breaths before returning to the center and repeating on the opposing side.

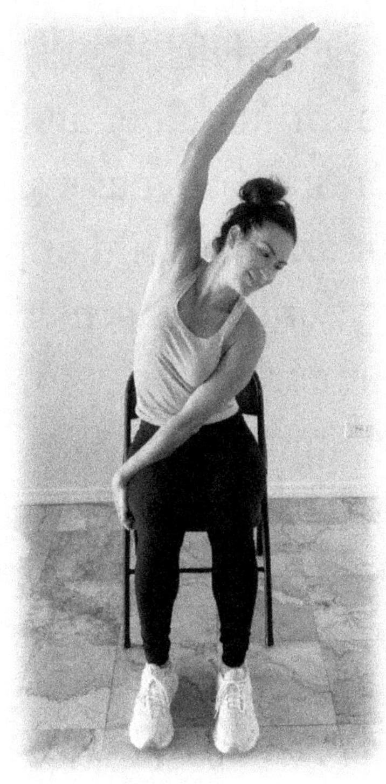

Chair Half Moon Pose

Benefits:

- Stretches and expands the hips, increasing mobility and decreasing stiffness.
- Uses core muscles to maintain balance and stability while developing the abdominals and obliques.

- Lengthens the spine and extends the side body, increasing spinal flexibility and movement.

Seated Tree Pose Variation:

i. Sit tall in your chair, feet level on the floor, hands resting on your thighs.

ii. Lift one foot off the floor and press the sole on the inner calf or thigh of your standing leg.

iii. Extend your arms upward or place your hands together at your heart's center.

iv. Engage your core muscles to stay balanced and stretch your spine.

v. Hold the posture for a few breaths before releasing and repeating on the opposing side.

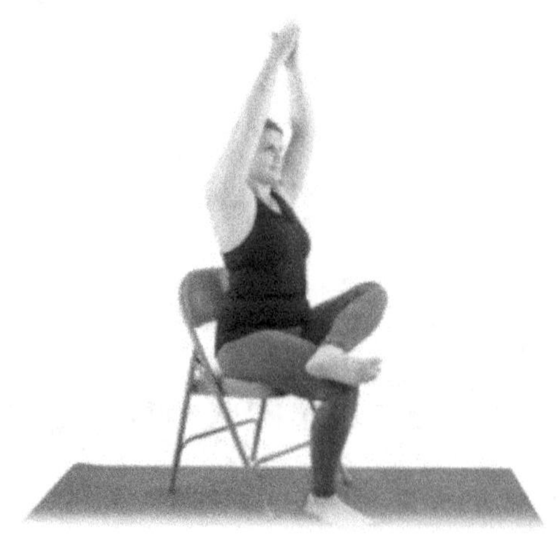

Seated Tree Pose Variation

Benefits:
- Tests balance and stability while increasing proprioception and coordination.
- Engages the standing leg muscles, such as the quadriceps, hamstrings, and calf.
- Mental attention and concentration are required, since they promote mindfulness and mental clarity.

Seated Eagle Pose Variation:
i. Begin by sitting tall in your chair, feet flat on the floor, hands resting on your thighs.
ii. Cross one thigh over the other, then bring your knees together and stack them on top of each other.
iii. Wrap the upper foot around the calf of the standing leg, if feasible, or just push the foot against the shin for support.
iv. Extend your arms out to the sides at shoulder height, then cross them in front of your body, elbows bent and palms together.
v. Engage your core muscles to stay balanced and deepen the stretch over your shoulders and upper back.

vi. Hold the posture for a few breaths before releasing and repeating on the opposing side.

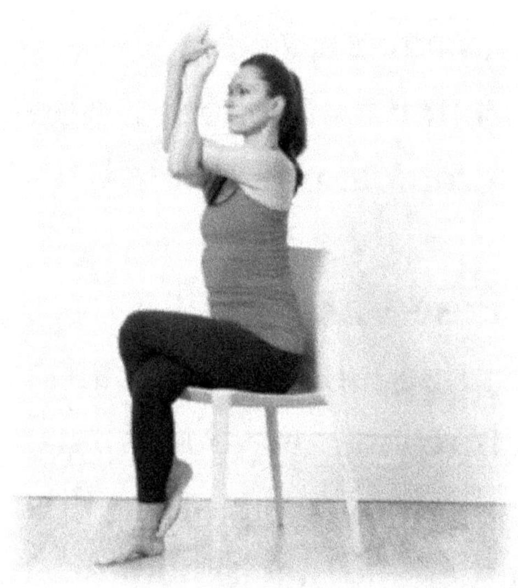

Seated Eagle Pose Variation

Benefits:

- **Shoulder Mobility:** Stretches and expands the shoulders, easing stress and tightness in the upper back and neck.

- **Hip Mobility:** Exercises the muscles of the hips and glutes, increasing mobility and flexibility.

- **Improves attention:** Tests concentration and attention, encouraging awareness and mental presence.

Seated Warrior II Variation:

i. Sit at the front edge of your chair, feet hip-width apart and firmly planted on the floor.

ii. Extend one leg straight behind you, toes pointing forward, heel elevated.

iii. Bend your front knee, ensuring it is exactly over your ankle, and move your body to the side.

iv. Extend your arms to the sides, shoulder height, and reach through your fingertips.

v. Engage your core muscles to maintain your spine and extend the stretch into your inner thigh and hip.

vi. Hold the posture for a few breaths, feeling the strength and stability develop in your legs and core.

vii. Repeat on the other side.

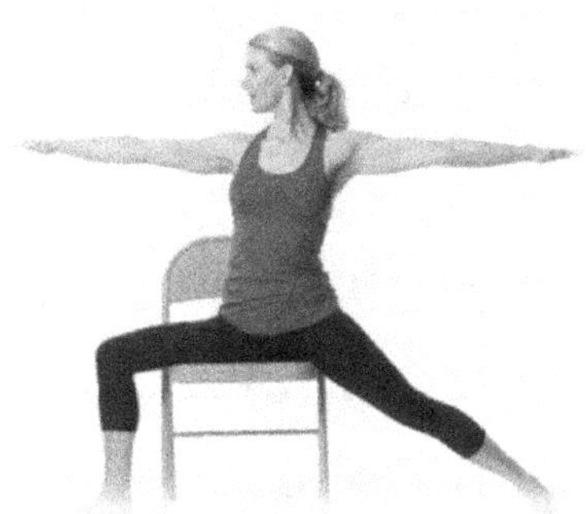

Benefits:

- This posture develops the leg muscles, particularly the quadriceps, hamstrings, and calves, resulting in increased lower body strength and stability.
- The Warrior II version opens up the hips and increases flexibility in the hip joints, decreasing stiffness and pain.
- Balancing in this posture involves focus and concentration, which can assist in sharpening mental awareness and improve mindfulness.

Seated Warrior III, Twist Variation:

i. Begin by sitting tall in your chair, feet flat on the floor, hands resting on your thighs.

ii. Extend one leg straight back behind you, with your toes pointed and heel elevated.

iii. Lean forward slightly, stretching your arms forward at shoulder level and raising your extended leg to hip level.

iv. Rotate your body to one side, with your opposite hand on your outer thigh and your other arm reaching for the sky.

v. Engage your core muscles to keep your balance and deepen the twist in your spine.

vi. Hold the posture for a few breaths before releasing and repeating on the opposing side.

Benefits:

- This version works the core muscles to maintain balance and stability, strengthening the abs and obliques.
- The twisting action in this position improves spinal mobility and flexibility, improving good posture and lowering spinal tension.
- Twisting postures activate the abdominal organs, which improve digestion and promote cleansing.

Seated Pigeon Pose Variation:

i. Sit tall in your chair, feet level on the floor, hands resting on your thighs.

ii. Cross one ankle over the other knee to form a figure-four formation with your legs.

iii. Flex your upper foot to cushion your knee, then softly press down on the crossing knee to deepen the stretch.

iv. Engage your core muscles to maintain stability and stretch your spine.

v. Hold the posture for a few breaths to feel the stretch in your outer hip and glute muscles.

vi. Repeat on the opposing side to balance out the stretch.

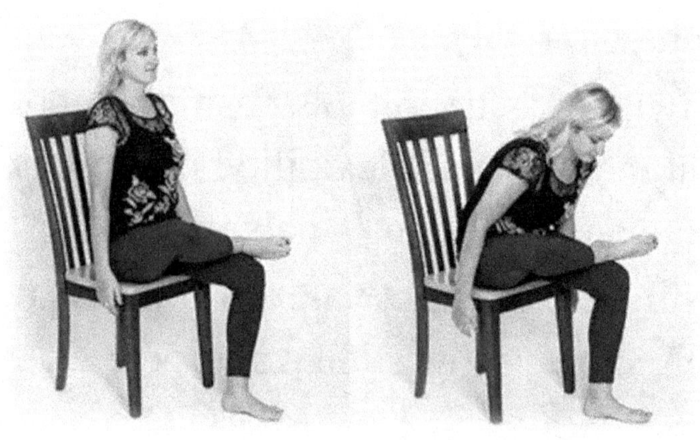

Seated Pigeon Pose Variation

Benefits:

- The seated pigeon posture variant opens the outer hip and glute muscles, improving hip mobility and decreasing hip tension.

- This position can assist relieve tension and stiffness in the hips and lower back, encouraging relaxation and stress reduction.
- By loosening up the hips and releasing tension in the lower body, the sitting pigeon pose variant can help with general posture and alignment.

Seated Crescent Lunge Pose Variation:

i. Sit tall in your chair, feet level on the floor, hands resting on your thighs.

ii. Extend one leg straight back behind you, with your toes pointed and heel elevated.

iii. Bend your front knee, ensuring it is exactly over your ankle, and raise your arms overhead.

iv. Engage your core muscles to maintain your spine and increase the stretch in your hip flexors and quads.

v. Hold the posture for a few breaths, feeling the strength and stability develop in your legs and core.

vi. Repeat on the opposite side to even out the strain and strengthen both sides of your body.

Benefits:

- This version works the leg muscles, particularly the quadriceps, hamstrings, and glutes, resulting in increased lower body strength and stability.
- The Crescent lunge position variant stretches the hip flexors, decreasing tension and increasing hip joint flexibility.
- The dynamic aspect of this posture can aid in increasing circulation and energy flow throughout the body, encouraging vitality and invigoration.

Seated Reverse Warrior Pose:

i. Begin by sitting tall in your chair, feet flat on the floor, hands resting on your thighs.

ii. Extend one leg straight out to the side, with your toes pointed and heel raised.

iii. Lean to the opposite side, raising your arm and bending your body toward the extended leg.

iv. Maintain your balance by engaging your core muscles and lengthening your side body.

v. Hold the posture for a few breaths, feeling the strain on the side of your body.

vi. Repeat on the opposite side to even out the strain and strengthen both sides of your body.

Benefits:

- The seated reverse warrior pose stretches the side body, particularly the intercostal and ribcage muscles, resulting in increased flexibility and ease of movement.

- This position expands the chest and lungs, enhancing respiratory function and encouraging deeper breathing.

- Seated reverse warrior position may boost energy and improve mood, making it an excellent pose to practice when feeling fatigued or sluggish.

Common problems and challenges with balance

Common issues and problems connected to balance, especially among seniors, might include:

Fear of Falling: This is perhaps the most common anxiety. Previous falls or near-falls might increase a person's fear of falling again, forcing them to limit their activities and movements to avoid prospective mishaps.

Loss of Mobility: As people age, their mobility may gradually deteriorate owing to causes such as joint stiffness, muscular weakening, and reduced flexibility. Reduced mobility might make it difficult to carry out daily tasks, leading to emotions of frustration and reliance.

Impaired Proprioception: Proprioception is the body's capacity to detect its location in space. Age-related alterations in proprioception can make it difficult to maintain balance and coordinate movements, increasing the risk of falling. Muscle weakness, particularly in the lower body and core, can impair stability and balance, making people more likely to fall.

Impaired Vision: Visual impairments, such as poor depth perception or limited peripheral vision, can impair balance and spatial awareness, increasing the risk of trips and falls.

Medication Side Effects: Certain drugs, notably those used to treat chronic diseases, may cause dizziness, sleepiness, or light-headedness, which can impair balance and coordination.

Chronic health issues: Chronic health issues, such as arthritis, Parkinson's disease, or peripheral neuropathy, can impair balance and movement, making it more difficult to maintain equilibrium.

Environmental Factors: Uneven surfaces, inadequate lighting, congested rooms, and a lack of handrails or grab bars can all increase the risk of falling, especially for people who have balance disorders.

Anxiety and Stress: Anxiety and stress can worsen feelings of instability and impair concentration, potentially compromising balance and coordination.

Foot Problems: Conditions such as foot discomfort, bunions, or neuropathy can impair balance and cause changes in stride and posture.

Cognitive Decline: Conditions such as dementia or Alzheimer's disease can impair spatial awareness, decision-making, and reaction times, increasing the risk of falling.

Deconditioning: Long periods of inactivity or sedentary behavior can cause muscular atrophy and diminished strength, jeopardizing stability and balance.

Vertigo, characterized by a sense of spinning or dizziness, can impair balance and coordination and may be caused by inner ear problems or vestibular diseases.

Nutritional Deficiencies: Insufficient consumption of certain nutrients, such as vitamin D or calcium, can weaken bones and muscles, reducing overall stability and raising the risk of falling.

Environmental Changes: Changes in the home environment, such as rearranged furniture, new barriers, or slick surfaces, might interrupt familiar movement patterns and impair balance and mobility.

Footwear Issues: Ill-fitting or improper footwear, such as shoes with worn-out soles or high heels, can impair stability and increase the risk of slipping and falling.

Lack of Confidence: Previous falls or near-misses might undermine confidence in one's ability to maintain balance, causing uncertainty and avoidance of specific activities or motions.

How to overcome typical issues associated with balance

Here are some tips and strategies for overcoming typical problems and challenges connected to balance: Participate in fall prevention programs or seminars that provide information on balance, strength training, and home safety adjustments.

Regular physical activity: Engaging in regular physical activity such as balancing exercises, strength training, and flexibility exercises, can help increase muscular strength, coordination, and stability.

Consider Tai Chi or Yoga: Both are good for improving balance, flexibility, and awareness, lowering the chance of falling.

Use Assistive Devices: Canes, walkers, or grab bars can give support and stability, especially in areas where falls are more common.

Wear Proper Footwear: To increase stability and minimize the chance of slips and falls, choose for supportive, well-fitting footwear with non-slip soles.

Address Vision Problems: Schedule regular eye exams and swiftly address any vision issues. Provide appropriate illumination throughout the home, particularly in places prone to falls.

Medication Management: Consult with a healthcare professional about any potential side effects that might impair balance or induce dizziness. Carefully follow the directions for your medicine.

Maintain a Healthy Diet: To maintain general strength and stability, consume a well-balanced diet rich in minerals needed for bone and muscular health, such as calcium, vitamin D, and magnesium.

Home Safety Modifications: Make changes to the home environment to lessen fall hazards, such as clearing clutter, fastening carpets, installing handrails and grab bars, and upgrading lighting.

Stay Hydrated: Drink enough water throughout the day to prevent dehydration, which can compromise balance and cognitive function.

Mindfulness Practices: Use mindfulness practices like deep breathing, meditation, or visualization to alleviate stress and anxiety, which can affect balance and attention.

Build Confidence: progressively push yourself to participate in activities that demand balance and coordination, beginning with little steps and progressively increasing difficulty as your confidence builds.

Seek Professional Help: Consult with healthcare specialists, physical therapists, or occupational therapists for specialized assessments, assistance, and suggestions based on your unique requirements and concerns.

Chapter 4: Chair Yoga for Flexibility and Mobility

Flexibility is the capacity of joints and muscles to move through their whole range of motion without discomfort or stiffness. It includes the flexibility of muscles, tendons, and ligaments, which allows for fluid movement and better posture. Mobility, on the other hand, refers to a wider range of motion, including the capacity to conduct useful motions like walking, bending, and reaching. Flexibility and mobility work together to build physical independence and quality of life, allowing seniors to go about their daily activities with ease and comfort.

Maintaining flexibility and mobility as we age is critical to our general health and well-being. Flexible muscles and joints promote appropriate alignment, lowering the likelihood of injury and discomfort. Improved mobility enables elders to carry out everyday duties independently, instilling a feeling of autonomy and confidence. Furthermore, flexibility and mobility help to improve posture, circulation, and joint health, increasing overall vitality and quality of life.

As we progress through this chapter, you may recognize familiar yoga positions and practices from other sections of the book. I want to reassure you that this repetition is deliberate and good. Each position performs numerous functions and provides distinct benefits, depending on the environment and emphasis of the practice. Returning to familiar positions with new eyes and an open mind allows you to gain deeper knowledge, perfect your technique, and feel the intricacies of each movement.

So, whether you've tried yoga before or not, I encourage you to approach each posture with inquiry and kindness. Accept the chance to investigate the tiny differences, see how your body responds, and develop a stronger connection between breath, movement, and consciousness. Remember that the essential meaning of yoga is not learning difficult positions, but rather the path of self-discovery and self-care.

As we continue our examination of chair yoga for flexibility and mobility, let us appreciate the freedom of movement that awaits us. Together, we'll discover how yoga may alter your life by increasing flexibility, mobility, and vitality.

Improving Flexibility and Mobility with Chair Yoga

"Enhancing Flexibility and Mobility through Chair Yoga" is a component that delves into the mild yet effective chair yoga practices for developing flexibility and mobility, with a focus on seniors over the age of 60. Chair yoga is a modified approach to conventional yoga postures, making them more accessible to people with limited mobility or physical impairments. We'll use accessible yoga postures and mindful movements to maximize your range of motion, enhance joint flexibility, and promote overall physical well-being.

Chair Yoga: A Path to Greater Freedom.

Chair yoga is a unique and accessible way to improve flexibility and mobility, making it an excellent practice for seniors of all ages and fitness levels. Individuals who use a chair for support can safely and comfortably do yoga postures that might otherwise be difficult or unattainable owing to physical constraints.

Chair yoga, with regular practice, helps to lengthen and stretch muscles, release tension in the body, and increase circulation—all of which lead to greater flexibility and mobility. Furthermore, chair yoga's conscious awareness creates a deeper connection between body and breath, promoting a sensation of comfort and relaxation that allows for more range of movement.

Exploring Gentle Yoga Poses

We'll go over a few mild yoga positions that are ideal for sitting or using a chair for support. These poses target certain parts of the body that are prone to stiffness and tightness, such as the spine, hips, shoulders, and legs. By gently stretching and moving these regions, you'll gain flexibility, less pain, and better overall mobility.

Each yoga position, from moderate twists and side stretches to forward bends and backbends, has its own set of advantages for increasing flexibility and mobility. With assistance on optimal alignment and adaptations to meet individual needs, you'll be able to explore your entire range of motion while being comfortable and safe in your chair.

By approaching movement with awareness and intention, you'll learn to move with more comfort and fluidity, while respecting your body's natural rhythms and limitations. With persistent practice, you'll progressively increase your range of motion, relieve tension, and rediscover the joy of easy movement.

Embrace the Journey

As we grow and learn more about improving flexibility and mobility with chair yoga, I want you to approach each practice with curiosity, compassion, and an open heart. Accept the chance to experience new experiences, uncover hidden strengths, and develop a stronger connection with oneself. Remember that the way to improve flexibility and mobility is about accepting the journey of self-discovery and self-care rather than striving for perfection.

Here are some chair yoga positions that promote mobility and flexibility:

Seated Cat-Cow Stretch:

i.   Sit tall on your chair, feet flat on the floor.
ii. Inhale while arching your back and lifting your chest (Cow Pose).

iii. Exhale as you circle your spine and lower your head forward (cat pose).

iv. Repeat for a few breaths.

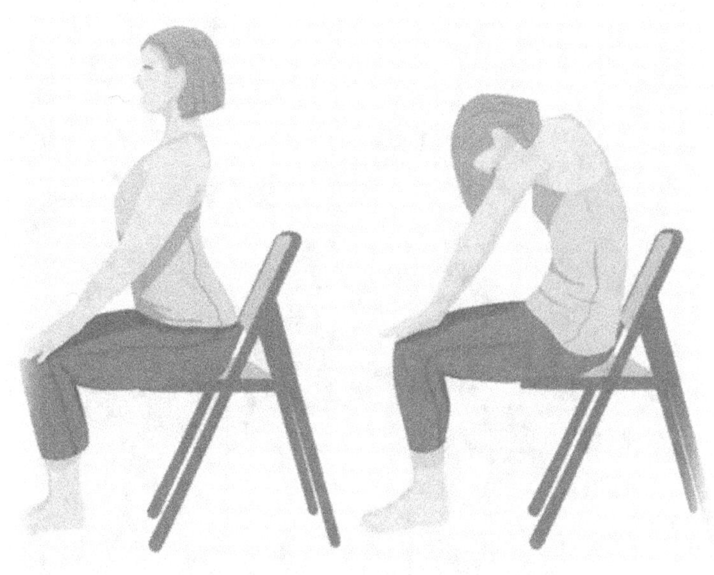

Seated Cat-Cow Stretch

Benefits:

- Improves spinal flexibility and mobility.
- Reduces stress in the back and neck muscles.
- Promotes improved posture and spinal alignment.

Seated Forward Fold:

i. Sit forward in the chair, feet hip-width apart.

ii.   Inhale to stretch the spine, then exhale to bend forward from the hips and reach for your feet or shins.

iii.   Hold for a few breaths before gently returning to an upright posture.

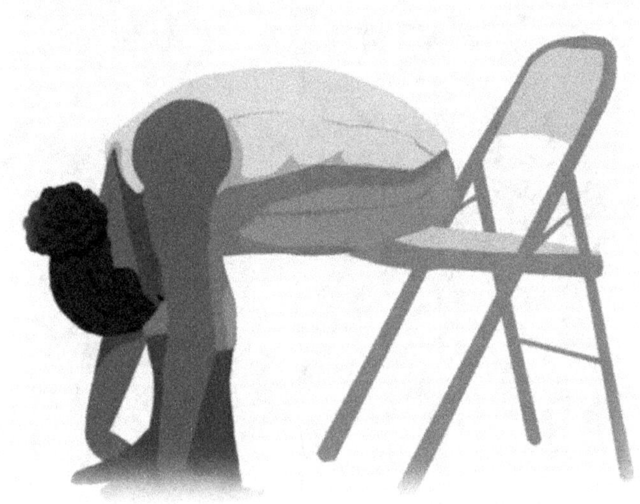

Seated Forward Fold

Benefits:

- Stretches the hamstrings, calves, and lower back.
- Increases flexibility in the spine and hips.
- Promotes relaxation and stress reduction.

Seated Twist:

i.   Sit tall, feet flat on the floor.

ii. Inhale to stretch your spine, then exhale to rotate
your body to the right, resting your left hand on
the outside of your right leg and your right hand on
the back of the chair.

iii. Hold for a few breaths before repeating on the
opposite side.

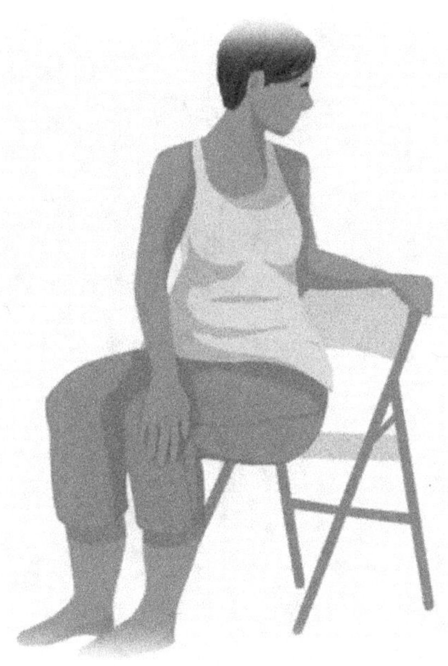

Seated Twist

Benefits:

- Enhances spinal mobility and flexibility.
- Stretches the back muscles and massages the
  organs.
- Promotes digestion and cleansing.

Seated Side Stretch:

i. Sit upright on your chair, feet flat on the floor.

ii. Inhale to stretch the spine, then exhale to extend your right arm above and bend to the left.

iii. Hold for a few breaths and then swap sides.

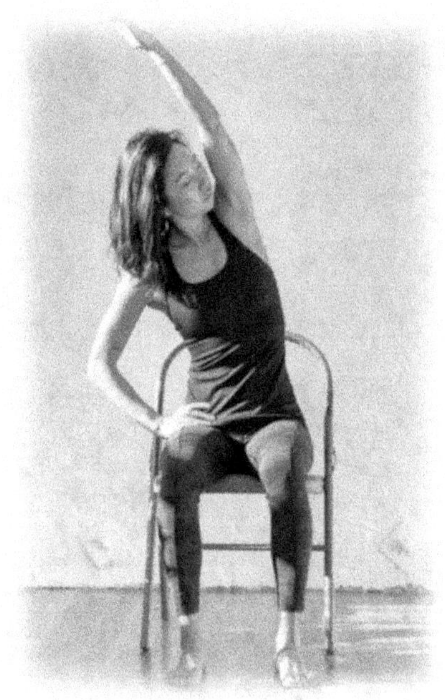

Seated Side Stretch

Benefits:

- Stretches both sides of the body, including the intercostal muscles.

- Increases spinal and shoulder flexibility.
- Releases stress in the ribs and waist.

Seated Knee to Chest Stretch:

i. Sit tall, feet flat on the floor.

ii. Lift one knee to your chest and wrap your hands around it.

iii. Hold for a few breaths and then swap legs.

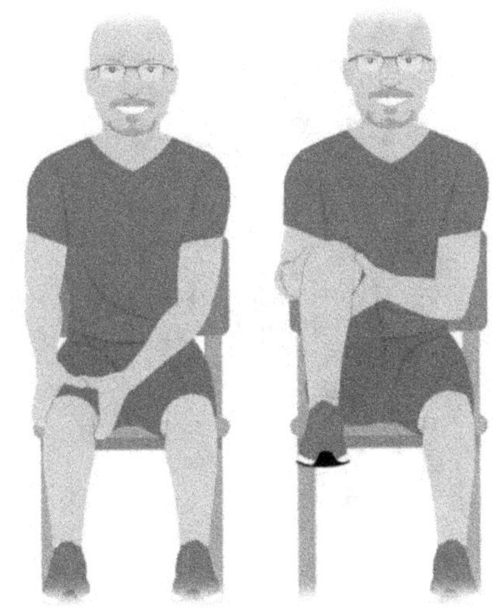

Seated Knee to Chest Stretch

Benefits:

- Stretches your hips, glutes, and lower back.
- Increases hip flexor flexibility and minimizes hip tightness.
- Relieves lower back pain and stiffness.

Seated Figure Four Stretch:

  i. Sit tall, feet flat on the floor.

  ii. Cross your right ankle across your left leg and flex your right foot.

  iii. Lean gently forward, keeping your spine straight.

  iv. Hold for a few breaths and then swap sides.

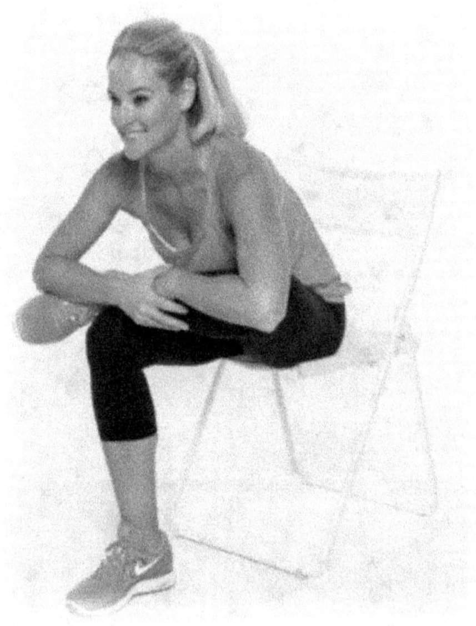

Seated Figure Four Stretch

Benefits:

- Stretches the outside hips and glutes.
- Enhances hip mobility and flexibility.

- Reduces stress and stiffness in the hips and lower back.

Seated Shoulder Opener:

i. Sit tall, feet flat on the floor.
ii. Interlace your fingers behind your back, straighten your arms, and raise your chest.
iii. Hold for several breaths before releasing.

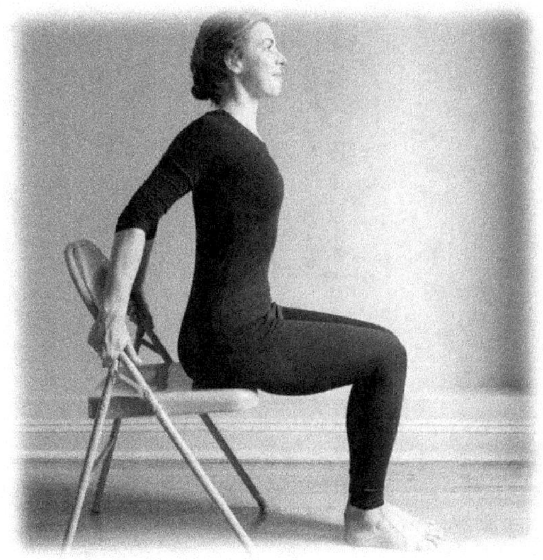

Seated Shoulder Opener

Benefits:

- opens the chest and shoulders.
- Stretches the front shoulders and chest muscles.

- Improves posture and reduces tension in the upper body.

Seated Ankle Circles:

i.   Sit tall, feet flat on the floor.

ii. Lift one foot off the ground and spin your ankle in circles, first in one direction, then the other.

iii. Repeat on the opposite side.

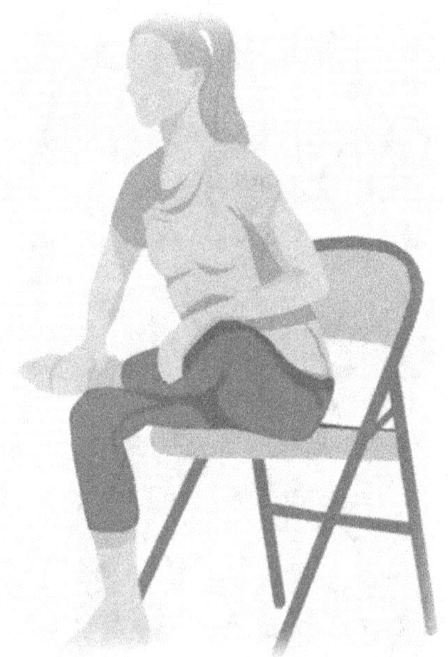

Seated Ankle Circles

Benefits:

- Improves ankle mobility and flexibility.
- Improves foot circulation and minimizes ankle stiffness.

- Helps to prevent ankle injuries and improves balance.

Seated Extended Side Angle Pose:

i.   Sit at the front edge of your chair, feet wide apart.

ii. Extend your right leg to the side while maintaining the left foot firmly planted.

iii. Reach your right arm down to your right shin or the floor, then extend your left arm above.

iv. Keep your torso looking forward and stretch your side body.

v.   Hold for a few breaths and then swap sides.

Benefits:

- Stretches the side body, which includes the obliques and intercostal muscles.
- Increases hip and shoulder flexibility.
- Enhances balance and stability.

Seated Pigeon Pose:

i.   Sit tall, feet flat on the floor.

ii. Cross your right ankle across your left leg and flex your right foot.

iii. Keep your spine straight and slowly tilt forward from the hips.

iv. Hold for a few breaths, experiencing a stretch in your outer hip and glutes.

v. Repeat on the opposite side.

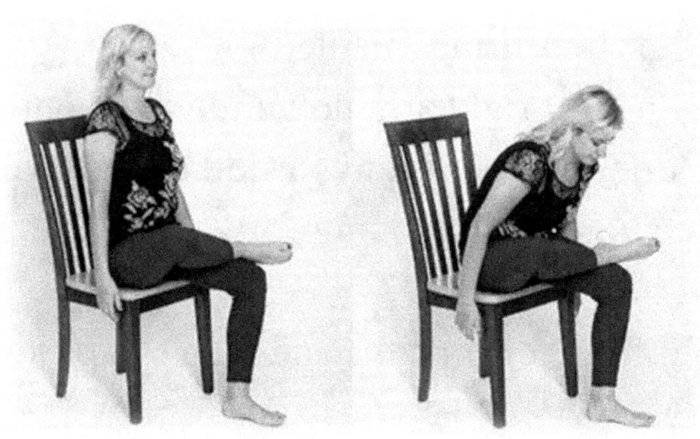

Seated Pigeon Pose

Benefits:

- Stretches the outside hips and glutes.
- Reduces stress and stiffness in the hips and lower back.
- Enhances hip mobility and range of motion.

Seated Spinal Twist:

i. Sit tall, feet flat on the floor.

ii. Inhale to extend your spine; exhale to rotate your body to the right.

iii. Place your left hand outside your right knee and your right hand on the back of the chair.

iv. Maintain a relaxed posture with your shoulders and spine stretched.

v. Hold for a few breaths and then swap sides.

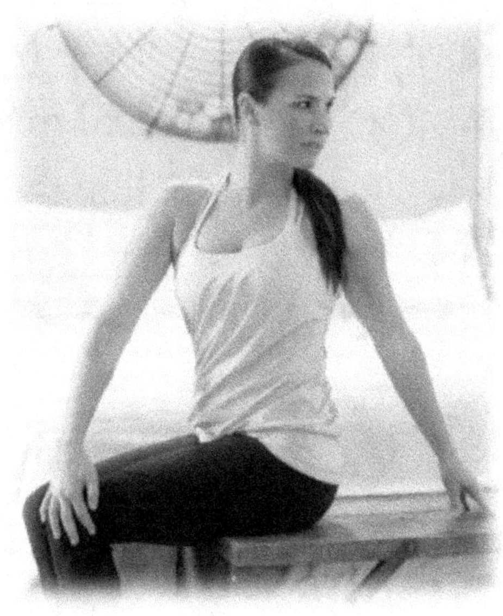

Seated Spinal Twist

Benefits:

- Enhances spinal mobility and flexibility.
- Promotes digestion and cleansing.

- Lower back discomfort is relieved by releasing muscular tension.

Seated Butterfly Stretch:
  i.   Sit tall, the soles of your feet together and knees out to the sides.
  ii. Hold your feet or ankles with your hands.
  iii. Gently push your knees down towards the floor to expand your hips.
  iv. Maintain a stretched spine and relaxed shoulders.
  v.   Hold for a few breaths, feeling the stretch in your inner thighs.

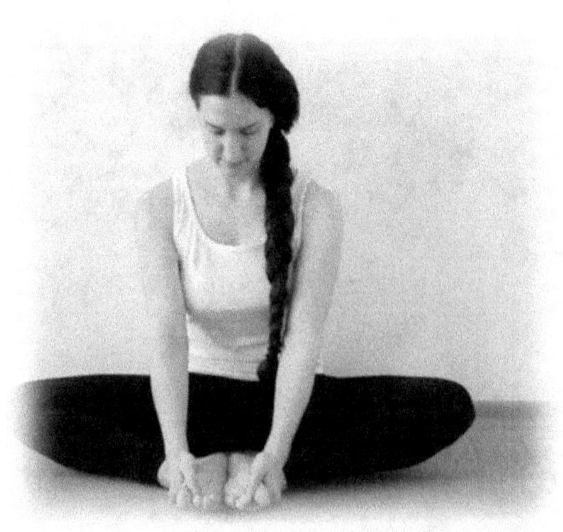

Seated Butterfly Stretch

Benefits:

- Stretches the inner thighs and groin muscles.
- Increases hip and pelvic flexibility.
- Reduces stress and stiffness in the hips and lower back.

Seated Shoulder Stretch:

i. Sit tall, feet flat on the floor.

ii. Reach your right arm across your chest and use your left hand to gently press it closer to your body.

iii. Maintain a comfortable posture with your shoulders and spine upright.

iv. Hold for a few breaths and then swap sides.

Benefits:

- Reduces stress and stiffness in the shoulders and upper back.
- Enhances shoulder mobility and range of motion.
- Lowers the risk of shoulder injuries and encourages proper posture.

Seated Hamstring Stretch:

i. Sit tall, legs straight out in front of you.

ii. Flex your feet and bend forward from the hips, reaching toward the toes.

iii. Keep your spine straight and your shoulders relaxed.

iv. Hold for a few breaths, feeling a stretch at the back of your legs.

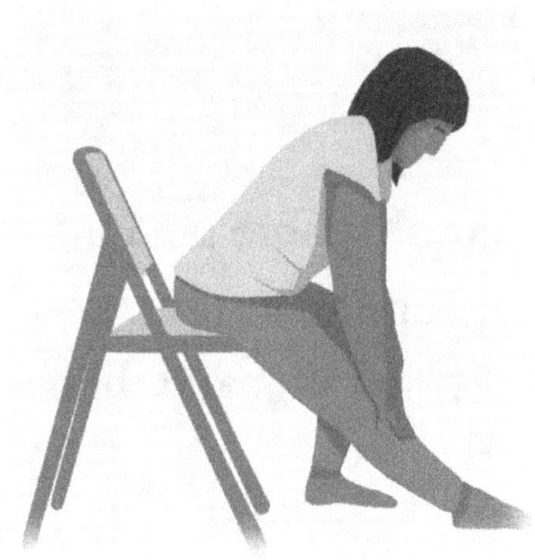

Seated Hamstring Stretch

Benefits:

- Stretches the calf and hamstring muscles.
- Increases flexibility in the legs and lower back.
- Reduces tightness and stiffness in the back of the legs.

Gentle Stretching Routines to Improve Range of Motion

Stretching is a crucial part of any workout routine, particularly for seniors who want to maintain or enhance their range of motion. Gentle stretching techniques can assist in promoting flexibility, reduce stiffness, and improve general mobility, allowing seniors to move more comfortably and easily during their daily activities.

In this part, we'll look at a variety of moderate stretching exercises that are especially intended to target important muscle groups and increase the range of motion. These exercises are safe, effective, and appropriate for people of all fitness levels, including seniors with restricted mobility and flexibility. These moderate stretching exercises will help you reach your goals of reducing joint stiffness, improving posture, and increasing general flexibility.

Each stretching practice will target various parts of the body, such as the neck, shoulders, back, hips, and legs. You may either do the entire program or choose particular stretches based on your requirements and interests. Remember to listen to your body and move gently and deliberately during each stretch, avoiding any movements that create pain or discomfort.

Here are some moderate stretching practices for seniors to increase their range of motion:

Neck Stretch:

i. Sit tall on your chair, feet flat on the floor.

ii. Gently tilt your head to the right, bringing your ear near your shoulder.

iii. Hold for 15-30 seconds and then swap sides.

iv. Repeat 2-3 times per side.

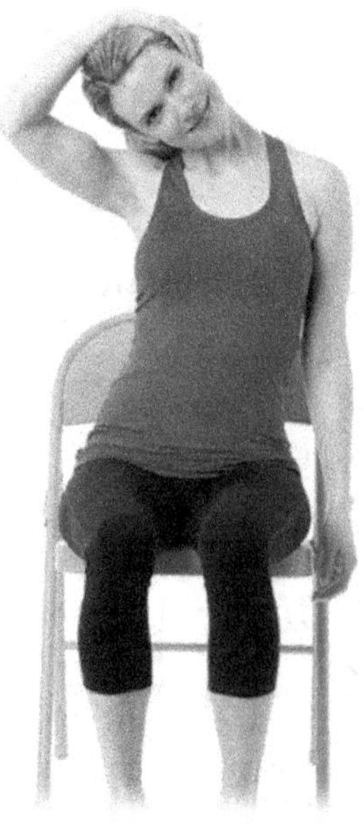

Neck Stretch

Benefits:

- Reduces stress and stiffness in the neck muscles.

- Improves cervical flexibility and range of motion.
- Reduces symptoms of neck discomfort, stiffness, and headaches.
- Promotes relaxation and decreases stress in the upper body.
- Improves posture and alignment by reducing tension in the neck and shoulders.

Shoulder Roll:

i. Sit tall, arms relaxed at your sides.
ii. Slowly move your shoulders forward in a circular manner.
iii. Repeat 5-10 times, then reverse direction and roll your shoulders backward.

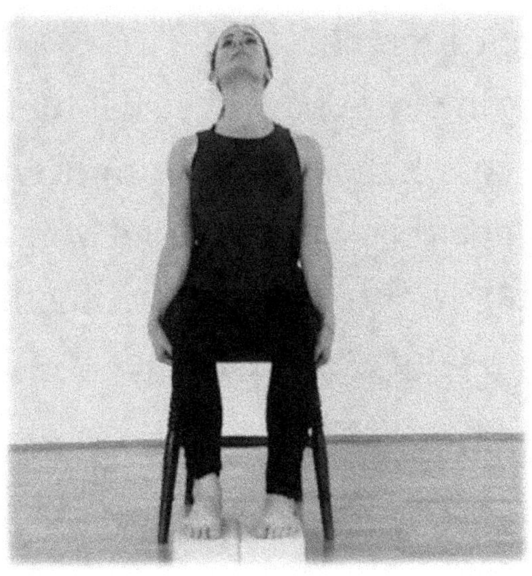

Benefits:

- Helps to relieve stress and stiffness in the shoulders.
- Enhances shoulder mobility and range of motion.
- Reduces pain caused by stiff shoulder muscles.
- Promotes relaxation and decreases stress in the upper body.
- Can help prevent or relieve symptoms of shoulder impingement and other shoulder-related problems.
- Increases circulation to the shoulders, improving overall shoulder health and function.

Upper Back Stretch:
  i.   Sit tall on your chair, feet flat on the floor.
 ii.   Clasp your hands together in front of you, round your upper back, and extend your arms forward.
iii.   Hold for 15-30 seconds, feeling the stretch between your shoulder blades.
iv.   Repeat 2–3 times.

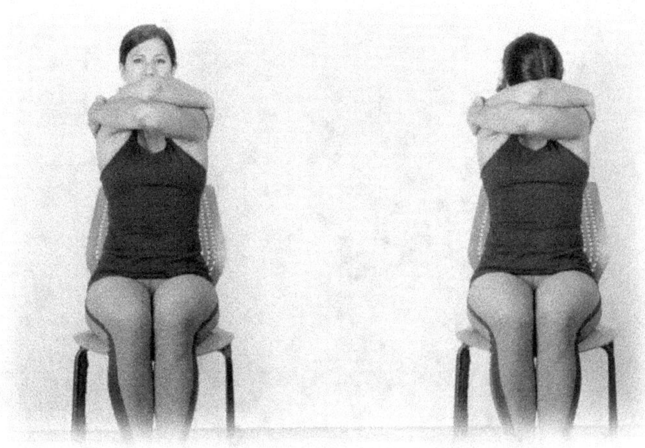

Upper Back Stretch

Benefits:

- Reduces stress and stiffness in the upper back muscles.
- Improves posture by expanding the chest and shoulders.
- Reduces pain caused by bad posture and prolonged sitting.

Chest Opener:

i.   Sit tall, feet flat on the floor, hands clasped behind your back.

ii. Gently press your shoulder blades together and raise your chest to the ceiling.

iii. Hold for 15-30 seconds and then release.

iv. Repeat 2–3 times.

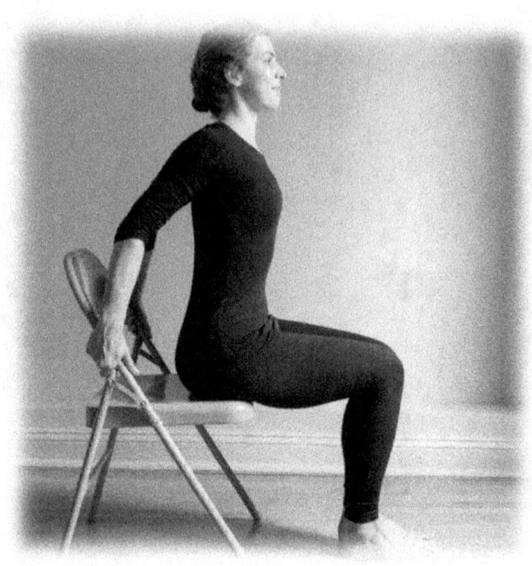

Benefits:

- Hunching or slouching can cause tightness in the chest muscles, thus this stretch helps.
- Improves posture by preventing forward rounding of the shoulders.
- Expands the chest cavity, allowing for deeper breathing and greater lung capacity.

Seated Forward Fold:

i. Sit forward in the chair, with your feet hip-width apart.

ii. Inhale to stretch your spine and exhale to bend forward from the hips.

iii. Reach your hands towards your feet or shins while maintaining your back straight.

iv. Hold for 15-30 seconds, feeling the stretch in your hamstrings and lower back.

v. Repeat 2–3 times.

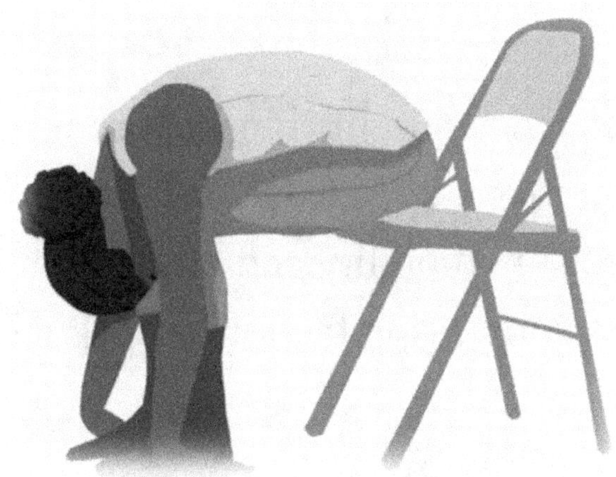

Seated Forward Fold

Benefits:

- Stretches the hamstrings, calves, and lower back.
- Relieves spinal tension and promotes relaxation.
- Reduces hip and lower body stiffness and increases range of motion.

Hip Flexor Stretch:

i. Sit tall, feet flat on the floor.

ii.   Extend your right leg forward, then lay your left ankle on your right knee.

iii. Lean slightly forward while maintaining your back straight, until you feel a stretch in your left hip.

iv.   Hold for 15-30 seconds and then swap legs.

v.   Repeat 2-3 times per side.

Benefits:

- Relieves tension in the hip flexor muscles, which might shorten due to extended sitting.
- Enhances hip mobility and range of motion.
- Reduces soreness in the lower back and hips.

Seated Hamstring Stretch:

i.   Sit tall, with your legs straight out in front of you.

ii.   Flex your feet and bend forward from the hips, reaching toward the toes.

iii. Maintain a straight back and prevent curving the spine.

iv.   Hold for 15-30 seconds until you feel a stretch in the back of your legs.

v.   Repeat 2–3 times.

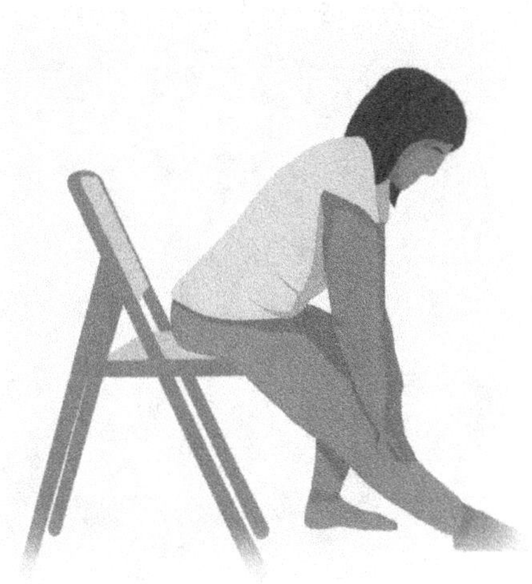

Seated Hamstring Stretch

Benefits:

- Stretches the hamstring muscles, which can become stiff due to prolonged sitting or lack of mobility.
- Increases flexibility and range of motion in the hamstrings and lower body.
- Lowers the likelihood of hamstring injuries while improving total leg function.

Ankle circles:

i. Sit tall, feet flat on the floor.

ii. Lift one foot off the ground, then gradually spin your ankle in a circular motion.

iii. Repeat 5–10 times in each direction, then move to the opposite foot.

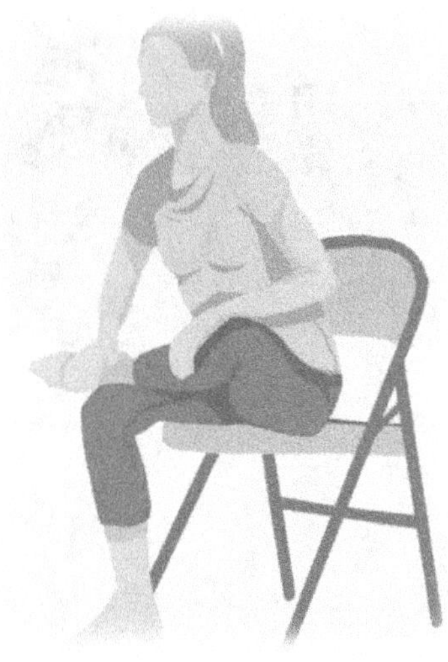

Ankle circles

Benefits:

- Increases ankle mobility and flexibility.
- Improves circulation in the feet and ankles.
- Helps to avoid ankle stiffness and lowers the chance of injury.

Seated Spinal Twist:

i. Sit tall, feet flat on the floor.

ii. Inhale to extend your spine; exhale to rotate your body to the right.

iii. Place your left hand outside your right knee and your right hand on the back of the chair.
iv. Hold for 15 to 30 seconds, experiencing a mild twist in your spine.
v. Repeat on the opposite side.

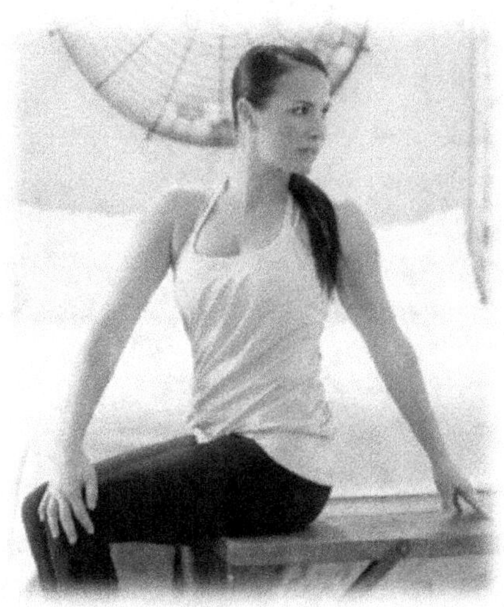

Seated Spinal Twist

Benefits:

- Enhances spinal mobility and flexibility.
- Releases tension in the spine and back muscles.
- Massaging the internal organs promotes digestion and cleansing.

Seated Side Bend:

i. Sit tall, feet flat on the floor, arms at your sides.

ii.   Inhale to stretch your spine and exhale to raise your right arm above.

iii. Lean to the left and feel a stretch on the right side of your body.

iv.   Hold for 15-30 seconds and then swap sides.

v.   Repeat 2-3 times per side.

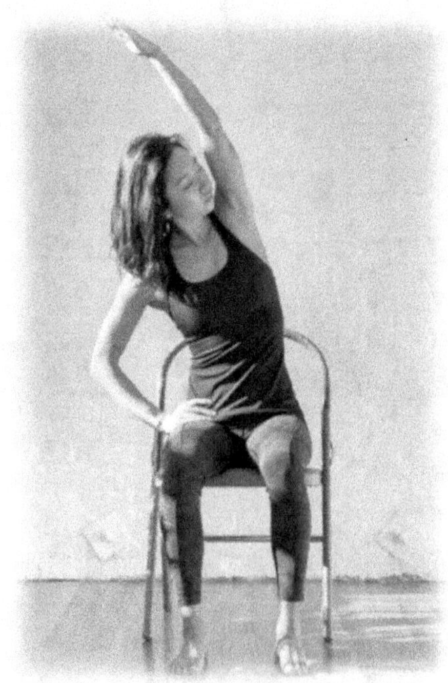

Seated Side Bend

Benefits:

- Stretches the side body, which includes the obliques and intercostal muscles.

- Increases lateral flexibility and range of motion in the spine.
- Reduces stress in the shoulders and ribcage.

Seated quadriceps stretch:

i. Sit tall, feet flat on the floor.
ii. Grab your left ankle with your left hand and slowly pull the heel towards your glutes.
iii. Keep your knees together and your torso upright.
iv. Hold for 15-30 seconds and then swap legs.
v. Repeat 2-3 times per side.

Benefits:

- Stretches the quadriceps muscles, which can become stiff due to prolonged sitting or lack of mobility.
- Quadriceps and hip flexors benefit from increased flexibility and range of motion.
- Reduces the likelihood of knee and hip problems while improving total leg function.

Seated Calf Stretch:

i. Sit tall, feet flat on the floor.
ii. Stretch your right leg forward and flex your foot.

   iii.   Reach your hands towards your right toes, feeling the stretch in your leg.
   iv.   Hold for 15-30 seconds and then swap legs.
   v.   Repeat 2-3 times per side.

Benefits:

- Stretches the calf muscles, which can get stiff after standing or walking.
- Increases ankle flexibility and range of motion.
- Reduces calves' pain and the danger of calf injuries.

Seated Wrist Stretch:

   i.   Sit up straight with your arms out in front of you at shoulder height.
   ii.   Flex your wrists so that your fingers point to the ceiling.
   iii.   Gently push down on the back of your hands with your opposing hand.
   iv.   Hold for 15-30 seconds, feeling the stretch in your wrists and forearms.
   v.   Repeat 2–3 times.

Benefits:

- Reduces strain and stiffness in the wrists and forearms.
- Increases wrist mobility and flexibility.
- Lowers the likelihood of repetitive strain injuries like carpal tunnel syndrome.

Seated Inner Thigh Stretch:

i. Sit tall, feet flat on the floor, knees bent.

ii. Place the soles of your feet together and let your knees fall to the sides.

iii. Use your hands to gently press your knees to the floor.

iv. Hold for 15-30 seconds, feeling the stretch in your inner thighs.

v. Repeat 2–3 times.

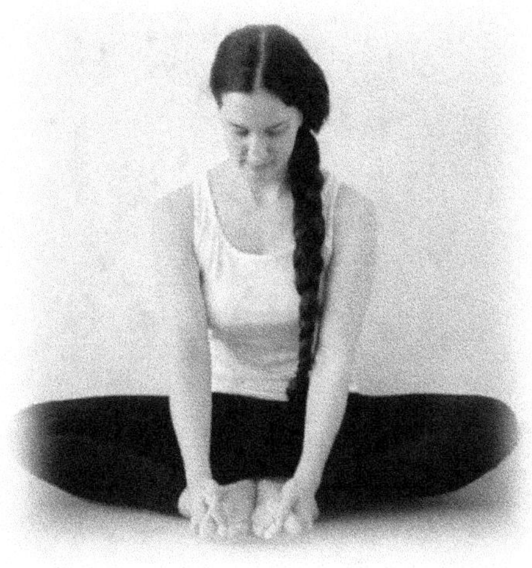

Benefits:

- Stretches the inner thigh muscles (adductor).
- Enhances hip mobility and flexibility.
- Reduces the likelihood of groin strains while improving total leg function.

Seated Side Neck Stretch:

i. Sit tall, shoulders relaxed, spine stretched.
ii. Drop your right ear towards your right shoulder, and feel a stretch down the left side of your neck.
iii. Hold for 15-30 seconds and then swap sides.
iv. Repeat 2-3 times per side.

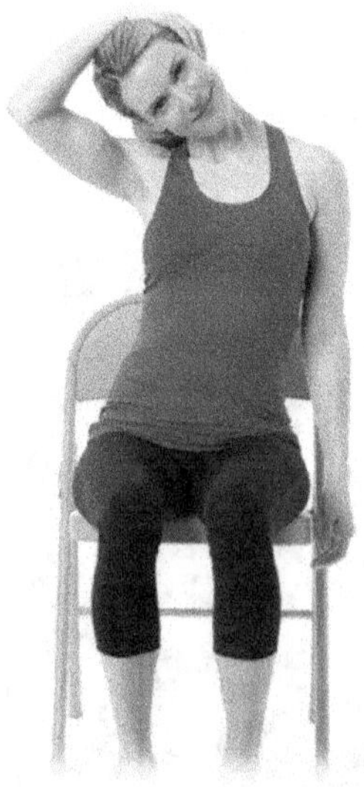

Seated Side Neck Stretch

Benefits:

- Reduces stress and stiffness in the neck muscles.
- Enhances neck mobility and flexibility.
- Reduces symptoms of neck discomfort, stiffness, and headaches.

Techniques to relieve joint stiffness and pain

Joint stiffness and discomfort may have a significant influence on seniors' everyday life, making ordinary movements such as walking, reaching, and even sitting hard. However, chair yoga offers powerful ways of relieving joint stiffness and discomfort, enhancing general mobility and quality of life.

Gentle joint mobilization exercises:

Begin by gently moving the joints through their complete range of motion, beginning with the neck and progressing down to the ankles.

To avoid strain or discomfort, move slowly and with control.

Increase flexibility and lubricate your joints to minimize stiffness and increase movement.

Breathing Techniques For Relaxation:

Deep breathing exercises can help to relax and alleviate stress in the body.

Practice diaphragmatic breathing by inhaling deeply with your nose and expelling completely through your mouth.

Concentrate on releasing any tension or stiffness in the muscles, particularly near the joints.

Mindfulness Meditation for Pain Management:

Engage in mindful meditation activities to increase awareness of bodily sensations, including regions of discomfort or pain.

Use visualization methods to visualize the breath moving into and out of the afflicted joints, providing warmth and relaxation.

Accept the sensations you have without judgment, enabling your body to feel more at peace and comfortable.

Heat Therapy For Joint Relief:

Apply heat treatment to the afflicted joints to relax muscles, enhance blood flow, and relieve pain and stiffness.

Use heating pads, warm towels, or heat packs to gradually warm the region for 15-20 minutes at a time. To avoid burns or injury, use caution while applying high heat or leaving heat sources unattended.

Chair Yoga Positions for Joint Flexibility:
Incorporate mild chair yoga postures that are particular to the problematic joints, such as wrist circles, ankle rolls, and shoulder shrugs.
Slow, deliberate motions can help to gradually stretch and strengthen the muscles that surround the joints.
Pay attention to any feelings you feel during the postures, and make any necessary changes to guarantee your comfort and safety.

Range of motion exercises:
Perform modest range-of-motion exercises for each joint, moving it through its entire range of motion without creating pain.
Begin with modest motions, gradually increasing the range as permitted.
Focus on fluid motions to keep the joints lubricated and flexible.

Joint-specific stretches:
Stretches that are specific to a joint's range of motion and function should be used.

For example, execute wrist flexion and extension stretches to relieve wrist stiffness, or knee flexion and extension exercises to increase knee mobility.

Hold each stretch for 15-30 seconds, then repeat multiple times on each side.

Hydrotherapy:

Use hydrotherapy, such as warm water treatment or swimming, to relieve joint stiffness and discomfort.

The buoyancy of water relieves stress on joints while providing resistance for strengthening.

Improve joint mobility by engaging in modest aquatic workouts or just moving and stretching in the water.

Joint Supportive Nutrition:

Maintain a well-balanced diet high in nutrients that promote joint health, such as omega-3 fatty acids, antioxidants, and vitamins C and D.

Include foods like fatty fish, leafy greens, berries, nuts, and seeds in your diet to decrease inflammation and increase joint lubrication.

Stay hydrated by drinking enough of water throughout the day to keep your joints healthy and flexible.

Use of Assistive Devices:

Consider utilizing assistive equipment like canes, walkers, or braces to help support and stabilize your joints throughout daily tasks.

Ergonomic equipment and aids, such as cushioned handles or reachers, can help decrease joint strain and make activities simpler.

Consult a physical therapist or occupational therapist for suggestions on the best assistive devices for your requirements.

Chapter 5: Mindfulness and Stress Reduction

In today's fast-paced world, stress has become a constant companion for many people, particularly seniors. However, by practicing mindfulness, we may learn to negotiate life's problems with more ease and resilience.

Mindfulness is the discipline of remaining in the present moment without judgment or attachment to ideas or emotions. It entails being curious and open to our ideas, feelings, physiological experiences, and the environment around us. Mindfulness can help us achieve more clarity, relaxation, and general well-being.

In this chapter, we will look at the advantages of mindfulness for seniors, including how it may assist with stress, anxiety, and other mental health issues. We'll learn simple strategies and exercises that may be applied in everyday life to enhance relaxation and inner calm.

In addition, we will look at the science underpinning mindfulness and how it affects the brain and body.

Understanding the physiological and psychological principles behind mindfulness might help us appreciate its enormous influence on our health and happiness. Whether you're new to mindfulness or have been practicing for years, this chapter provides essential insights and skills to help you on your path to higher well-being.

Effects of Mindfulness on the Brain and Body

The benefits of mindfulness on the brain and body are varied and deep. Here are some major effects: Mindfulness has been shown to increase neuroplasticity, or the brain's ability to restructure itself by generating new neural connections. Regular mindfulness practice can cause anatomical changes in the brain, such as increased gray matter density in regions responsible for attention, emotion management, and memory.

Stress Reduction: Mindfulness activities, such as meditation and deep breathing exercises, stimulate the body's relaxation response, lowering the production of stress chemicals like cortisol and adrenaline. This can lead to lower perceived stress, less anxiety, and increased mood.

Mindfulness improves the brain's ability to regulate emotions by strengthening the prefrontal cortex, which is responsible for cognitive control and decision-making. It also decreases activity in the amygdala, the brain's fear region, resulting in improved emotional stability and resilience.

Improved Attention and Concentration: Studies have demonstrated that mindfulness training improves attentional control and sustained focus. Individuals who practice present-moment awareness can teach their brains to filter out distractions and stay focused on the work at hand.

Pain Management: Mindfulness-based therapies have been shown to reduce chronic pain by changing the brain's interpretation of pain signals. Mindfulness helps people adopt a non-reactive attitude toward pain, which reduces the emotional misery and suffering that comes with it.

Enhanced Immune Function: Evidence suggests that mindfulness techniques can improve immune function by lowering inflammation and increasing immune cell activity. This can contribute to increased resistance to infections and quicker recovery from sickness.

Improved Sleep Quality: Mindfulness practices, such as relaxation exercises and body scans, can help people relax and fall asleep. Mindfulness, which calms the mind and body, can help people sleep deeper and more soundly.

Greater Well-being: Mindfulness practice has been related to higher levels of subjective well-being and life satisfaction. Individuals who practice present-moment mindfulness and acceptance might enjoy more peace, satisfaction, and fulfillment in their lives.

Reduced Depression Symptoms: Mindfulness-based therapies have been proven to improve depression symptoms by encouraging a more balanced mood and reducing rumination, which is a prominent component of depressed thinking.

better Cognitive Function: Mindfulness techniques have been linked to better cognitive function, including memory, decision-making, and problem-solving abilities. Regular mindfulness practice may aid in preserving cognitive vibrancy and prevent age-related cognitive decline.

Mindfulness promotes resilience by helping people acquire more self-awareness, emotional control, and adaptive coping techniques. This resilience enables people to recover more rapidly from losses and obstacles, retaining a sense of calm in the face of adversity.

Better Relationships: Mindfulness can enhance interpersonal relationships by increasing empathy, compassion, and communication abilities. Individuals who practice present-moment mindfulness and nonjudgmental acceptance can improve their connections with others and develop more meaningful and harmonious relationships.

Reduced Risk of Cardiovascular Disease: Mindfulness practices have been linked to better cardiovascular health, such as lower blood pressure, lower heart rate, and increased blood flow. These physiological changes may help lower the risk of heart disease and stroke.

Enhanced Body Awareness: Mindfulness enables people to tune into their bodies and become more aware of bodily feelings including tension, pain, and discomfort. This increased bodily awareness enables improved self-care and proactive control of health concerns.

Mindfulness increases emotional intelligence by encouraging increased self-awareness, self-regulation, and empathy. Individuals who practice mindfulness are more capable of understanding and managing their emotions, as well as empathizing with the feelings of others.

Mindfulness promotes self-compassion by urging people to treat themselves with love, understanding, and acceptance. This self-compassionate attitude can buffer against negative self-judgment and self-criticism, leading to improved general well-being.

Mindfulness activities have been demonstrated to boost creativity by quieting the mind and cultivating open awareness. This mental clarity and openness can lead to creative thoughts and inventive problem resolution.

Chair Yoga Techniques for Stress Relief

Stress may be a serious worry for everyone, but it is more prevalent among seniors. Fortunately, chair yoga is an excellent stress-reduction technique because it combines easy motions and breathing exercises with the mindfulness and relaxation benefits associated with yoga. Let's go over some strategies you may utilize to alleviate stress using chair yoga.

Mindful breathing exercises:

Begin by sitting comfortably in your chair, feet flat on the floor, and hands resting on your thighs.

If you're comfortable, close your eyes or soften your focus, and take a few deep breaths in through your nose and out your mouth.

Concentrate your focus on the sensation of the breath as it enters and exits your body, noting the rise and fall of your chest or the expansion and contraction of your stomach.

Continue breathing deeply and regularly, allowing each breath to calm and relax your mind and body.

Counting your breaths can help you focus.

Chair Yoga Stretches:

Gently stretch and move the body to relieve tension and encourage relaxation. Focus on stress-prone parts of the body, such as the neck, shoulders, and upper back.

For example, shrug your shoulders up towards your ears before rolling them back and down in a smooth circular motion. Repeat numerous times, alternately rotating clockwise and counterclockwise.

You may also perform neck stretches by gently tilting your head to one side, bringing your ear closer to your shoulder, and holding for a few breaths. Repeat on the other side.

Guided Relaxation Meditation:

i. Close your eyes and direct your attention within, concentrating on the sensation of your breath and the rhythm of your heartbeat.

ii. Visualize yourself in a peaceful and beautiful setting, such as a quiet beach or a lush forest. Imagine yourself surrounded by warmth and comfort, utterly protected and relaxed.

iii. As you continue to breathe deeply and slowly, allow any thoughts or anxieties to melt away, leaving you peaceful and centered.

iv. Stay in this state of relaxation for as long as you choose, appreciating the sense of peace and calm that emerges.

Body Scan Meditation:
  i. Begin by focusing your attention on the sensations in your feet, noting any areas of tightness or discomfort.
  ii. Move your focus slowly up your body, assessing each portion for evidence of tension or stress and intentionally releasing any stiffness or holding.
  iii. Continue to work through each region of your body, beginning with your legs and hips and progressing to your abdomen, chest, arms, and lastly your head and neck.
  iv. With each breath, envision yourself releasing any physical or mental tension, allowing yourself to sink deeper into a state of calm and peace.

Seated Cat-Cow Stretch:
  i. Sit comfortably in your chair, feet flat on the floor, hands resting on your thighs.
  ii. Inhale as you arch your back, elevate your chest, and tilt your pelvis forward (Cow pose).
  iii. Exhale while rounding your back, lowering your chin to your chest, and pulling your belly button towards your spine (cat pose).

iv. Repeat this fluid action while breathing, alternating between arching and rounding your back to relieve spinal tension and promote relaxation.

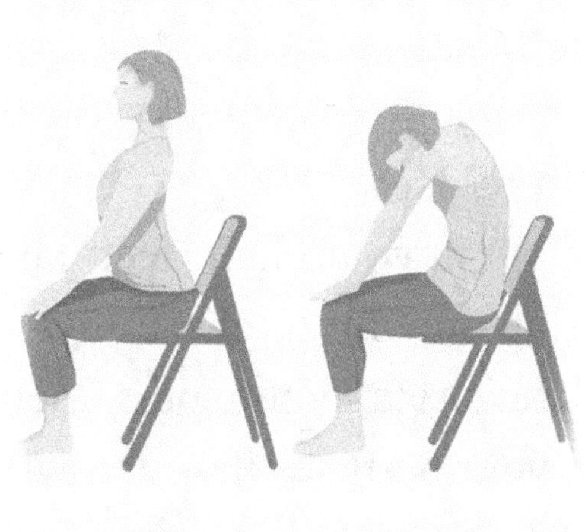

Seated Cat-Cow Stretch

Seated Forward Fold with Breathing Awareness:
  i. Sit at the front edge of your chair, feet hip-width apart and firmly planted on the floor.
 ii. Inhale as you extend your spine and raise your arms overhead.
iii. Exhale as you tilt forward at the hips, pushing your chest towards your thighs and allowing your arms to dangle lightly to the floor.

iv. Relax your neck and shoulders, and concentrate on the sensation of your breath flowing in and out of your body.

v. Hold the forward fold for a few breaths, experiencing a nice stretch in your hamstrings and lower back as any tension melts away with each exhalation.

Seated Twisting Pose:

i. Sit up straight in your chair, feet flat on the floor, hands resting on your thighs.

ii. Inhale as you stretch your spine, then exhale as you rotate your body to the right, with your left hand on the outside of your right leg and your right hand on the back of the chair.

iii. Maintain a long spine as you slowly twist, utilizing your breath to deepen the stretch with each exhalation.

iv. Hold the twist for a few breaths before inhaling to return to the center and repeating on the opposite side.

v. Twisting positions serve to relieve stress in the spine and massage the internal organs, encouraging relaxation and cleansing.

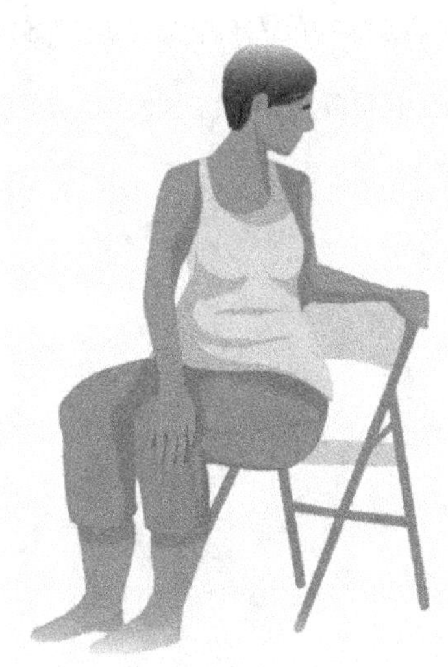

Seated Twisting Pose

Seated Eagle Arms Stretch:

i.   Sit comfortably in your chair, feet flat on the floor, arms at your sides.

ii. Inhale while reaching your arms out to the sides, shoulder height.

iii. Exhale and cross your right arm over your left, wrapping your forearms and palms together.

iv. Lift your elbows slightly and bring your shoulder blades down your back until you feel a stretch in your upper back and shoulders.

v.   Hold the stretch for a few breaths before releasing and repeating on the opposite side.

vi. The Eagle arms stretch relieves tension in the shoulders and upper back, fostering relaxation and comfort.

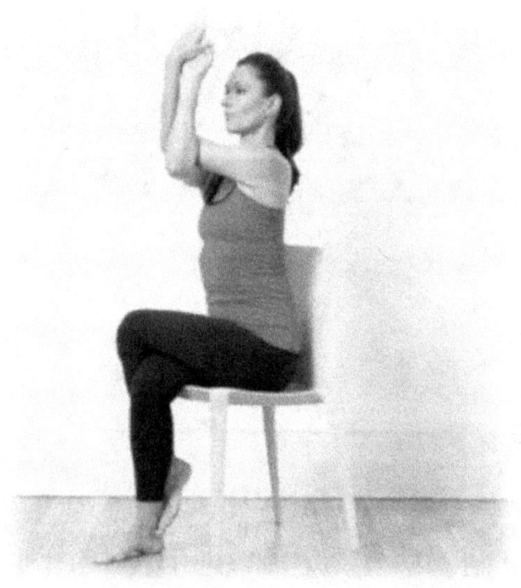

Seated Eagle Arms Stretch

Seated shoulder shrugs and rolls:
i. Sit comfortably in your chair, feet flat on the floor, hands resting on your thighs.
ii. Inhale while shrugging your shoulders up towards your ears, tightening the muscles in your shoulders and neck.
iii. Exhale to relieve tension, letting your shoulders sink down and back.

iv. Repeat this action many times, matching your breath with the movement, then switching directions to roll your shoulders forward and up, then back and down.

v. Shoulder shrugs and rolls relieve tension in the shoulders and neck, which promotes relaxation and reduces stress.

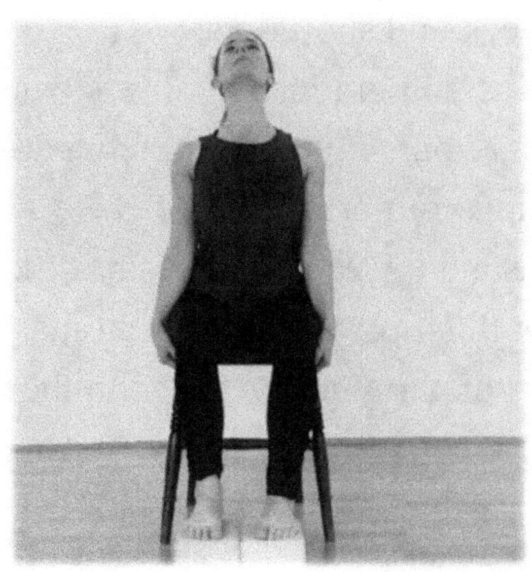

Seated shoulder roll

Seated Sun Salutation Variation:

i. Sit at the front edge of your chair, feet hip-width apart and hands resting on your thighs.

ii.   Inhale while raising your arms upwards and reaching tall through your fingertips.

iii.   Exhale as you bend forward at the hips, bringing your chest to your thighs and your hands to your feet.

iv.   Inhale to stretch your spine, then raise your hands halfway up to your shins or thighs.

v.   Exhale to fold forward again, relieving tension in your neck and shoulders.

vi.   Inhale as you gradually roll up to a sitting posture, stacking your spine one vertebra at a time and returning your arms overhead.

vii.   Exhale and lower your arms back to your sides.

viii.   Repeat this flowing movement many times, synchronizing your breath with the motion to induce relaxation and relieve tension in your body.

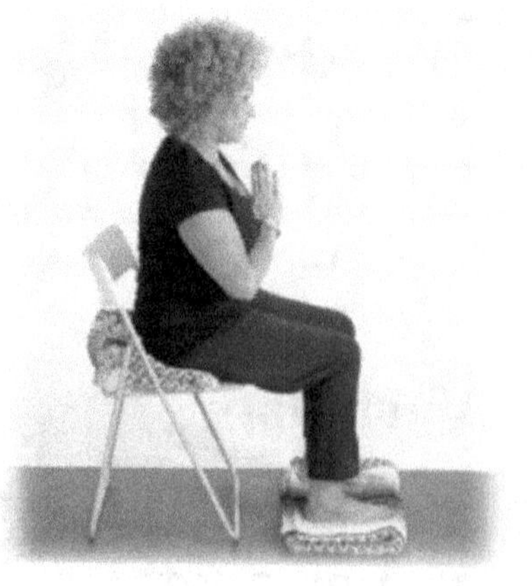
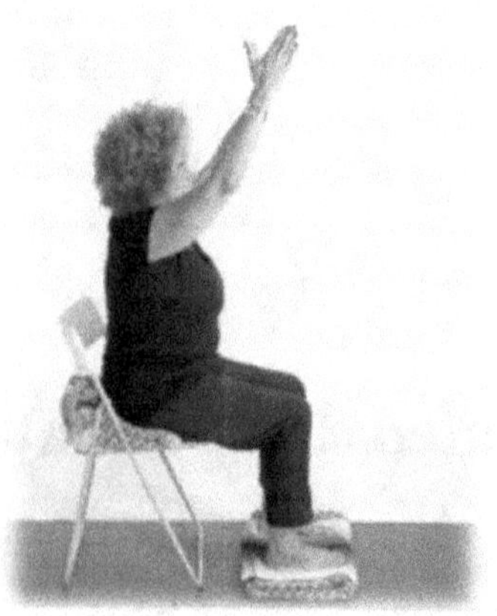

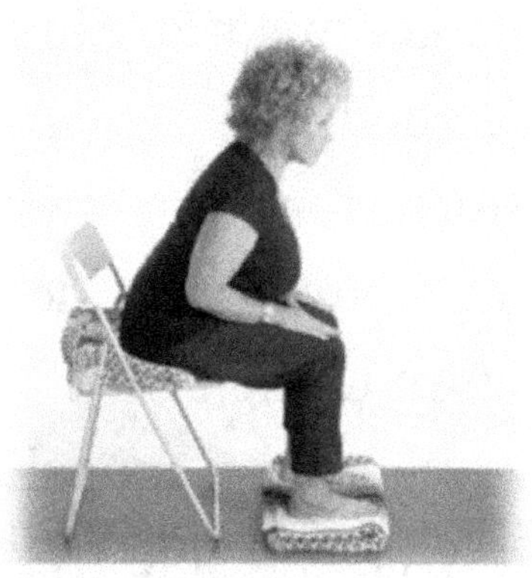

Seated Sun Salutation Variation

Seated Twist and Side Stretch:

i. Sit comfortably in your chair, feet flat on the floor, hands resting on your thighs.

ii. Inhale as you stretch your spine, then exhale as you rotate your body to the right, with your left hand on the outside of your right leg and your right hand on the back of the chair.

iii. Inhale to stretch your spine, then exhale to deepen the twist, gently moving your head to gaze over your right shoulder if comfortable.

iv. Hold the twist for a few breaths before inhaling and returning to the center.

v. Exhale while reaching your right arm up and across to the left, resulting in a side stretch through the right side body.

vi. Hold the stretch for a few breaths until you feel a mild opening in the right side ribs and waist.

vii. Inhale to return to the center, then repeat the twist and side stretch on the opposite side.

viii. This sitting twist and side stretch combo relieve tension in the spine and side body, encouraging relaxation and stress reduction.

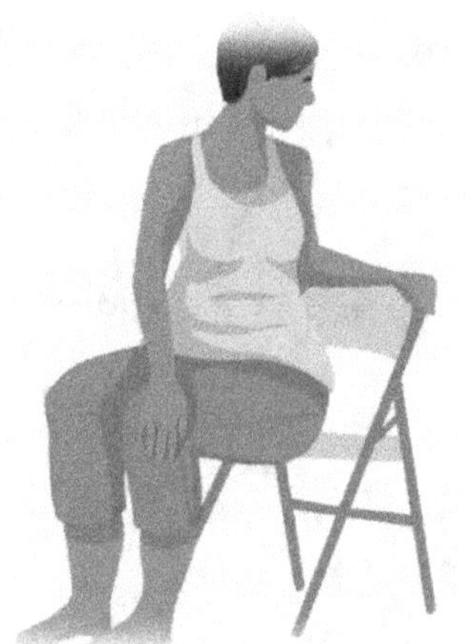 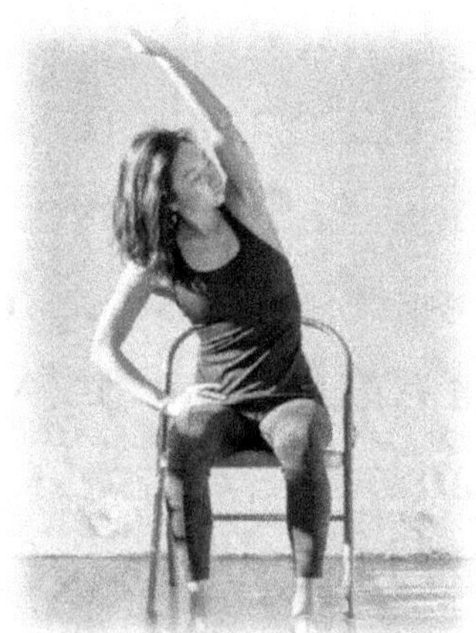

Seated Twist and Side Stretch

Seated Leg Extension and Forward Fold:

i. Sit up straight in your chair, feet flat on the floor, hands resting on your thighs.

ii. Inhale as you stretch your spine, then exhale as you extend your right leg out in front of you and flex your right foot.

iii. Inhale to extend your spine, then exhale to tilt forward at the hips, bringing your chest to your thigh and reaching your hands for your right foot.

iv. Hold the forward fold for a few breaths, feeling the stretch on the back of your right leg and hamstring.

v.   Inhale to return to a sitting position, then exhale to lower your right leg down.

vi. Repeat the leg extension and forward fold on the left side.

vii. This sitting leg extension and forward fold exercise stretches the hamstrings and promotes relaxation.

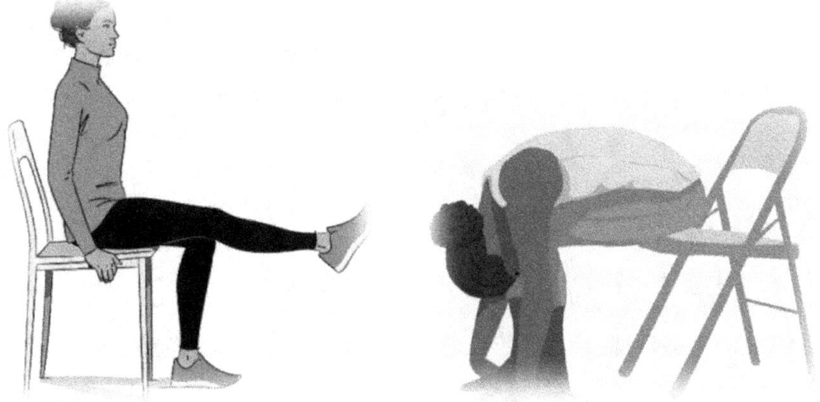

Seated Leg Extension and Forward Fold

Practices for Promoting Inner Peace and Relaxation

Finding moments of inner calm and relaxation might seem like a rare luxury in today's environment. However, chair yoga allows you to create a sanctuary of quiet inside yourself, regardless of where you are or what obstacles you are experiencing. In this part, we'll look at many activities that are expressly meant to promote inner calm and relaxation, allowing you to handle life's ups and downs with greater ease and grace.

Guided Relaxation Meditation:

i. Take a comfortable sitting position on your chair, feet flat on the floor and hands softly resting in your lap.

ii. Close your eyes if it is comfortable, or soften your look, and take a few deep breaths to center yourself.

iii. Begin to pay attention to your breath, noting the natural pattern of breathing and exhaling.

iv. As you continue to breathe deeply, envision a calm and beautiful setting in your mind, such as a quiet beach, a tranquil forest, or a snug mountain home.

v. Imagine yourself in this peaceful setting, surrounded by beauty and tranquillity, feeling entirely protected and at ease.

vi. Allow yourself to sink further into relaxation with each breath, letting go of whatever tension or worry you may be carrying.

vii. Stay in this deep relaxation state for as long as you choose, experiencing the sense of peace that comes over you.

Body Scan Meditation:

i. Begin by focusing your attention on your feet, noting any sensations of warmth, tingling, or heaviness.

ii. Move your attention slowly up your body, checking for signs of tension or discomfort and intentionally releasing any stiffness or holding.

iii. Take your time moving through each region of your body, starting with your feet and legs and progressing to your hips, tummy, chest, arms, and lastly your head and neck.

iv. With each breath, envision yourself releasing any physical or mental tension, allowing yourself to sink deeper into a state of calm and peace.

 v. Continue scanning your body from head to toe until you're entirely calm and at ease.

Loving-kindness Meditation:
  i. Sit comfortably in your chair and close your eyes. Take a few deep breaths to focus on yourself.

 ii. Bring to mind someone you care greatly about, whether it's a family member, friend, or pet, and see them in your mind.

iii. While focusing on this individual, quietly say the following sentences to yourself: "May you be happy, healthy, safe, and at peace."

iv. Continue to repeat these sentences, bringing love, compassion, and well-being to your loved one.

 v. After spending some time sending loving-kindness to this individual, gradually broaden your circle of compassion to include more loved ones, acquaintances, and even people you don't know directly.

vi. Finally, practice loving-kindness toward oneself, wishing yourself pleasure, health, safety, and tranquility.

vii. Sit with these sentiments of love and compassion for a few seconds, allowing yourself to soak up the warmth and shine of your loving-kindness.

Deep breathing exercises:

i. Sit comfortably in your chair, feet flat on the floor, hands resting on your thighs.

ii. Close your eyes if it's more comfortable, or soften your focus, and take a few deep breaths in through your nose and out your mouth.

iii. As you continue to breathe deeply, focus on the sensation of your breath going in and out of your body.

iv. Consider how your breath glides freely in and out, similar to the ebb and flow of the ocean tide.

v. Imagine inhaling serenity, tranquility, and relaxation, filling your body with light and pleasant energy.

vi. With each exhale, visualize yourself releasing tension, stress, and negativity, letting go of everything that is no longer useful to you.

vii. Continue to breathe deeply and rhythmically, allowing each breath to ground you in the present moment and promote inner calm and relaxation.

Progressive muscle relaxation:

i. Sit comfortably in your chair and close your eyes. Take a few deep breaths to focus on yourself.

ii. Begin by focusing your attention on your feet, then gradually tension the muscles in your feet and toes as you inhale.

iii. Hold the strain for a few seconds, then exhale as you release the tension entirely, allowing your feet to relax fully.

iv. Slowly work your way up your body, tensing and releasing each muscle group in turn, starting with your calves and ending with your face.

v. With each breath, the tension melts away, leaving you feeling thoroughly rested and at ease.

Guided Imagery Meditation:

i. Sit comfortably in your chair and close your eyes. Take a few deep breaths to focus on yourself.

ii.   Imagine yourself in a relaxing place of your choice, such as a rich garden, a peaceful alpine lake, or a quiet meadow.

iii. Immerse yourself in this fictional environment by exploring the sights, sounds, scents, and sensations that surround you.

iv.   Allow yourself to relax and unwind as you explore this tranquil setting, experiencing serenity and calm pour over you with each breath.

Affirmation Meditation:

i.   Choose a positive affirmation that speaks to you, such as "I am calm and centered," "I am worthy of love and happiness," or "I trust in the wisdom of the universe."

ii.   Sit comfortably in your chair and close your eyes. Take a few deep breaths to focus on yourself.

iii. With each inhale and exhale, repeat your selected affirmation, either silently or aloud, to enable the words to seep into your subconscious mind and promote a sense of calm and well-being.

Body Awareness Meditation:
i.   Sit comfortably in your chair and close your eyes. Take a few deep breaths to focus on yourself.
ii. Focus your attention on your physical body, noting any places of tension, discomfort, or pain.
iii. With each breath, give love and compassion to these regions, allowing them to soften and relax.
iv. Concentrate on the feelings in your body, noticing the tiny motions of your breath and the soft rhythm of your heartbeat.
v.   Continue to breathe deeply, feeling connected and harmonious with your body, knowing you are secure, protected, and truly loved.

Chapter 6: Chair Yoga for Specific Health Concerns

It is common for us to have certain health difficulties as we age, which can influence our physical, mental, and emotional well-being. Whether you are coping with chronic pain, managing a medical condition, or simply want to improve your general health, chair yoga provides a gentle and accessible approach to wellness that can be tailored to your specific requirements.

The activities included in this chapter are intended to help you on your road to better health and vitality by giving specific exercises and approaches to address prevalent health issues among seniors. Chair yoga, which mixes movement, breath, and mindfulness to promote healing and balance, can help manage arthritis and osteoporosis, relieve back pain, and improve heart health.

Throughout this chapter, you'll find a variety of chair yoga techniques designed to treat various health conditions. Each exercise is accompanied by detailed instructions and adaptations to guarantee accessibility for people of all skill levels and abilities. Whether you're new to yoga or an experienced practitioner, you'll discover useful techniques and insights to help you improve your health and well-being.

Always remember that the route to good health is unique to each individual. Listen to your body, respect your limitations, and go into your practice with an open mind and heart. You may build improved health, energy, and resilience at any age by dedicating yourself, being compassionate, and utilizing the transforming power of chair yoga.

Adapting Chair Yoga to Common Health Conditions

Chair yoga may be tailored to meet common health concerns for seniors, providing gentle and effective practices that promote healing, mobility, and general well-being. Each practice is tailored to meet the particular demands and problems of various health conditions, with changes and variations to provide accessibility and safety for practitioners of all levels.

Arthritis:

Chair yoga can help relieve stiffness, inflammation, and discomfort from arthritis. To develop flexibility and range of motion while minimizing pain, focus on mild joint motions and supported positions.

Osteoporosis:

Individuals with osteoporosis should avoid high-impact movements that increase the risk of fractures. Chair yoga offers a secure and supportive environment in which to strengthen bones and improve balance with modest weight-bearing postures and mindful movements.

Back pain:

Chair yoga can help relieve back pain and improve spinal health. Gentle stretches, twists, and strengthening exercises can help relieve stress, improve posture, and promote overall spine health.

Heart health:

Chair yoga promotes heart health by reducing stress, lowering blood pressure, and increasing circulation. Concentrate on soft motions that encourage relaxation and awareness, such as deep breathing exercises and restorative positions.

Diabetes:

Chair yoga's gentle motions and breathing methods can help manage blood sugar levels and increase insulin sensitivity. Gentle stretches and relaxation exercises can help relieve stress and increase general well-being.

Anxiety and Depression:

Chair yoga can help manage anxiety and depression by creating a safe and supportive environment to promote mindfulness, self-awareness, and emotional resilience. Gentle motions, deep breathing exercises, and guided meditation can help you relax and find inner peace.

Chronic Pain:

Chair yoga's moderate motions and relaxation techniques can reduce chronic pain and enhance quality of life. Gentle stretches, mindfulness techniques, and breathwork can help reduce tension, improve relaxation, and boost resilience in the face of pain.

Chair Yoga for Arthritis, Osteoporosis, And Diabetes

Living with arthritis, osteoporosis, or diabetes can bring unique physical and mental problems. From managing chronic pain and inflammation to navigating changes in mobility and energy levels, persons with these disorders typically seek safe and effective strategies to support their health and well-being. This is where chair yoga comes in.

Chair yoga is a moderate and accessible approach to movement and mindfulness that allows people with arthritis, osteoporosis, and diabetes to increase flexibility, strengthen bones, decrease stress, and manage symptoms of their diseases. Whether you have tight joints, weak bones, or fluctuating blood sugar levels, chair yoga provides a safe and supportive atmosphere that promotes healing and improves overall quality of life.

Let's have a look at some chair yoga techniques that are particularly developed to meet the requirements of those with arthritis, osteoporosis, and diabetes. From mild joint motions and breathing exercises to weight-bearing postures and mindful relaxation methods, each practice is meticulously designed to provide therapeutic benefits for the body, mind, and soul. Remember that chair yoga isn't about perfection or competitiveness as we go through these techniques together. It's about accepting yourself precisely as you are and treating your body's wisdom and limits with love and care. Whether you're a novice or an experienced practitioner, there's something for everyone to discover and appreciate.

Chair Yoga for Arthritis:

Arthritis is a prevalent ailment that causes joint inflammation and stiffness, resulting in discomfort and decreased movement. Chair yoga is a gentle and accessible technique to increase flexibility, decrease inflammation, and relieve arthritis-related suffering. Here are some chair yoga techniques particularly developed for those who have arthritis.

Gentle Joint Movements:

Start by sitting comfortably in a chair, feet flat on the floor.

Slowly and gently move each joint in your body through its whole range of motion, beginning with your fingertips and toes and gradually progressing to your shoulders and hips. Concentrate on calm, steady movements and avoid jerking or rapid actions that may aggravate pain.

Breathing Exercises:
Deep breathing techniques can help relieve stress and discomfort linked with arthritis. Close your eyes and take slow, deep breaths in through your nose and out through your mouth, aiming to fill your lungs with each inhalation and exhale.

Chair Yoga Poses:
Try moderate chair yoga poses that target areas of stiffness and discomfort in the body, such as sitting spinal twists, gentle forward folds, and supported backbends.

Use props like bolsters, blankets, or blocks to give extra support and comfort as required.

Chair Yoga for Osteoporosis:
Osteoporosis is defined by poor bone density and increased risk of fractures, especially in the spine, hips, and wrists. Individuals with osteoporosis can benefit from chair yoga by strengthening bones, improving balance, and lowering their risk of falling. Here are some chair yoga techniques particularly suited for those who have osteoporosis.

Weight-Bearing Postures: Include modest weight-bearing postures in your chair yoga practice to strengthen and increase bone density. Examples include sitting warrior poses, chair squats and gentle standing poses using the chair as support.

Balance Exercises: Balance exercises can help increase stability and minimize the chance of falling, which is especially important for people who have osteoporosis. Try sitting tree pose variants, leg lifts, and heel-toe rises while clutching the chair's back for support.

Mindful Movement: Practice mindful movement and body awareness to lessen the chance of injury and encourage safe, productive practice. Pay attention to your body's cues and avoid any actions or postures that produce discomfort or tension.

Chair Yoga for Diabetes:

Diabetes is a chronic illness that causes high blood sugar levels, leading to issues such as cardiovascular disease, nerve damage, and visual difficulties. Chair yoga can help manage this condition. Chair yoga can help control diabetes by encouraging relaxation, lowering tension, and boosting circulation. Here are some chair yoga techniques particularly created for those who have diabetes.

Deep Breathing: Deep breathing exercises can help manage blood sugar levels and insulin sensitivity by promoting relaxation and reducing tension. Take slow, deep breaths in through the nose and out through the mouth, taking your time to fully exhale and release any tension.

Gentle Stretching: Include gentle stretching movements in your chair yoga practice to promote circulation and flexibility. Focus on exercises that relieve tension and stiffness, such as sitting side stretches, neck rolls, and ankle circles.

Mindful Eating: Use mindfulness practices to build a healthy connection with food and regulate blood sugar levels. Pay attention to your body's hunger and fullness signs, and take each bite slowly and deliberately.

Pose and Modifications for Pain Relief and Rehabilitation

Now is the time to look at chair yoga postures and modifications that can help people with arthritis, osteoporosis, and diabetes manage their pain and recover. These practices are intended to offer gentle and effective motions that reduce discomfort, promote healing, and improve general well-being.

Seated Cat-Cow Stretch:

i. To do the Seated Cat-Cow Stretch, sit comfortably in a chair with your feet flat on the floor and hands resting on your thighs.

ii. Inhale as you arch your spine, raise your chest, and roll your shoulders back (Cow Pose).

iii. Exhale while rounding your back, lowering your chin to your chest, and bringing your belly button toward your spine (Cat Pose).

iv. Repeat this slow-flowing movement multiple times, matching your breathing with your motions.

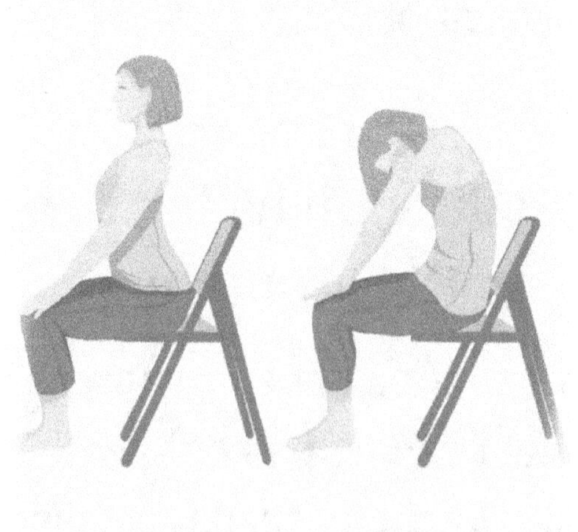

Seated Cat-Cow Stretch

Supported Side Bend:

i. Sit at the front edge of your chair, feet hip-width apart and firmly planted on the floor.

ii. Reach your right arm aloft and slowly lean to the left, with your left hand resting on the chair seat for support.

iii. Keep both sitting bones anchored while you lengthen the right side of your body, experiencing a mild stretch along the way.

iv. Hold the stretch for a few breaths before returning to the center and repeating on the opposing side.

Seated Pigeon Pose:

i. Sit at the front edge of your chair, feet hip-width apart, and firmly planted on the floor.

ii. Cross your right ankle over your left knee, and bend your right foot to cushion your knee.

iii. Maintain a long and tall spine as you softly tilt forward from your hips and lead with your chest.

iv. Hold the stretch for a few breaths, experiencing a deep stretch in the outer hip and glute muscles, before switching sides.

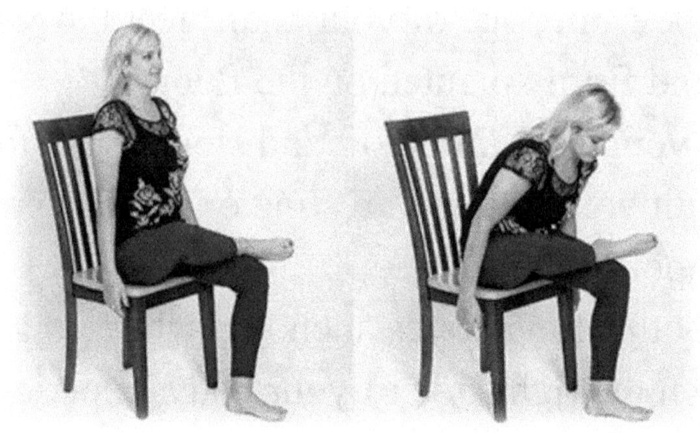

Seated Pigeon Pose

Supported Forward Fold:
  i. Sit at the front edge of your chair, feet hip-width apart and securely planted on the floor.
  ii. Inhale while sitting up straight.
  iii. Exhale while bending forward from your hips, keeping your spine long and your chest elevated.
  iv. Your hands can rest on your thighs, shins, or the floor, depending on your flexibility.
  v. Hold the stretch for several breaths until you feel a soft relaxation in your lower back and hamstrings.

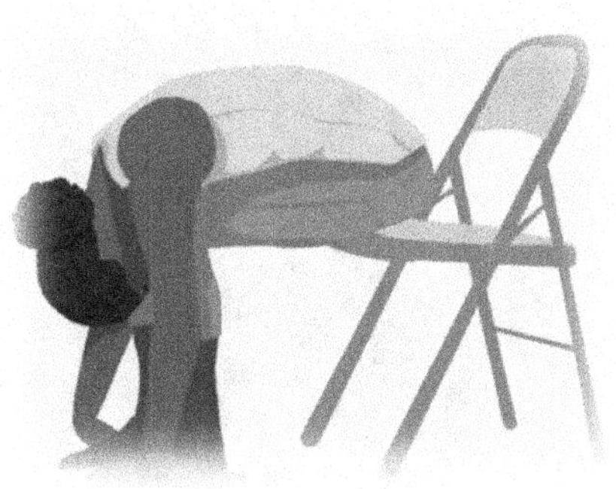

Chair Twist:

i.   Sit at the front edge of your chair, feet hip-width apart and firmly planted on the floor.

ii. Inhale while sitting up straight.

iii. Exhale while twisting to the right, with your left hand on the outside of your right leg and your right hand on the back of the chair.

iv. Maintain a long spine and relaxed shoulders as you deepen the twist with each exhalation.

v.   Hold the position for a few breaths before returning to the center and repeating on the opposing side.

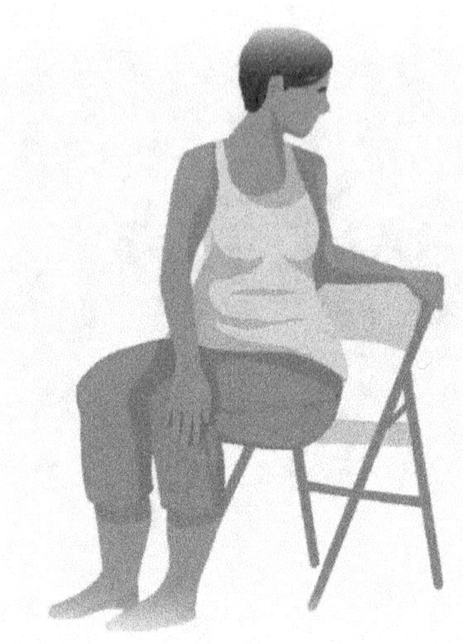

Chair Twist

Seated Forward Fold with Twist:

i. Sit at the front edge of your chair, feet hip-width apart and firmly planted on the floor.

ii. Inhale while sitting up straight.

iii. Exhale as you tilt forward from your hips, bringing your chest close to your thighs.

iv. Place your right hand on the outside of your left leg and your left hand on the back of the chair to provide support.

v. Deepen the stretch by slowly turning your torso to the left and letting your gaze follow.

vi. Hold the position for a few breaths, experiencing a slight stretch along the spine and outer hip, before switching sides.

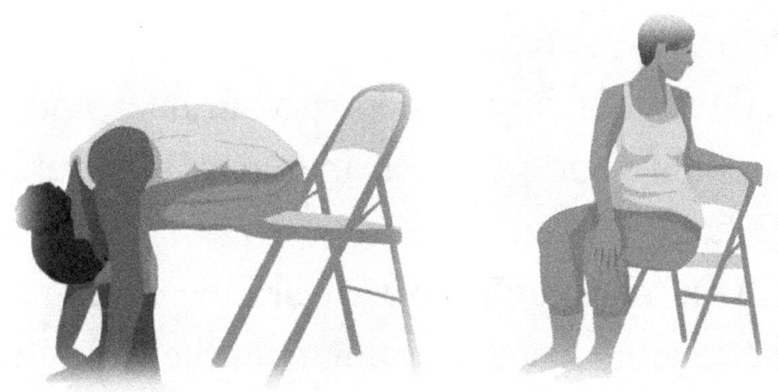

Seated Forward Fold with Twist

Seated Figure Four Stretch:

i. To perform the Seated Figure Four Stretch, sit at the front edge of your chair, feet hip-width apart, and firmly planted on the floor.

ii. Cross your right ankle across your left thigh, and bend your right foot to cushion your knee.

iii. Maintain a long and tall spine while softly pressing your right knee to the floor, experiencing a stretch in the outer hip and glute.

iv.   Hold the stretch for a few breaths before switching
      sides.

Seated Shoulder Opener:
  i.   To do the seated shoulder opener, sit comfortably
       with your feet flat on the floor.
 ii.   Interlace your fingers behind your back and
       straighten your arms to bring your shoulder blades
       together.
iii.   Lift your chest and stare toward the ceiling,
       experiencing a soft opening over the front of your
       chest and shoulders.
 iv.   Hold the stance for a few breaths before releasing
       and shaking out your arms.

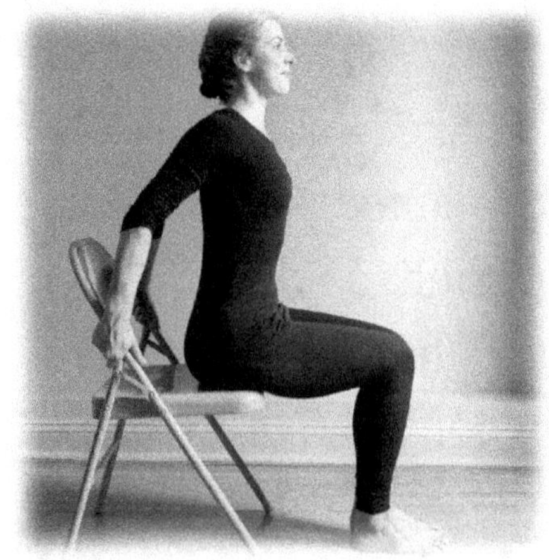

Seated Shoulder Opener

Seated Hip Opener:

  i.   Sit at the front edge of your chair, feet hip-width apart, and firmly planted on the floor.

 ii.   Place your right ankle on your left knee, flexing your right foot to protect it.

iii.   Maintain a long and tall spine while softly pressing your right knee to the floor, experiencing a stretch in the outer hip and glute.

 iv.   Hold the stretch for a few breaths before switching sides.

Seated Cat-Cow Twist:

  i.   Sit comfortably in your chair, feet flat on the floor.

 ii.   Inhale as you arch your spine, raise your chest, and roll your shoulders back (Cow Pose).

iii.   Exhale as you circle your spine, lowering your chin to your chest and moving your belly button closer to your spine (cat pose).

 iv.   Repeat the flowing action, twisting gently on either side as you arch and round your spine.

Seated Spinal Extension:

i. To do a seated spine extension, sit comfortably with your feet flat on the floor.

ii. Interlace your fingers behind your head and softly push your elbows backward.

iii. Lift your chest to the ceiling, expanding through the front of your body and stretching your spine.

iv. Hold the pose for a few breaths before releasing and returning to a neutral sitting position.

Chapter 7: 7-Day Chair Yoga Meal Plan

If you want to enhance your health and wellness with chair yoga, you need to think about both the exercises and your nutrition. A nutritious diet is vital for keeping your body strong and flexible. In this post, we will present a 7-day meal plan that supplements a chair yoga regimen, concentrating on natural foods and nutrient-dense meals.

As you've found throughout this book, chair yoga has several physical, mental, and emotional advantages. Chair yoga offers a comprehensive approach to fitness that goes beyond the mat, promoting flexibility and mobility while also lowering stress and increasing awareness. Nutrition, like yoga, is essential for fueling your body, maintaining your energy levels, and improving overall wellness.

This chapter will introduce you to a 7-Day Chair Yoga Meal Plan that is intended to supplement your yoga practice and help you feel your best from the inside out. Each day of the meal plan includes tasty and healthy foods carefully prepared to offer the nutrition your body requires to flourish. There are a range of selections to meet your taste preferences and nutritional demands, including vivid salads and robust soups, as well as healthful snacks and fulfilling dinners.

This meal plan, however, is more than simply a collection of recipes; it is a guide to developing a mindful and intuitive eating style that acknowledges your body's specific requirements while also supporting your health goals. Throughout the week, you'll be urged to pay attention to your body's hunger and fullness cues, appreciate each mouthful carefully, and replenish yourself with complete, nourishing foods that boost your energy and well-being.

Whether you want to improve your chair yoga practice, manage chronic health concerns, or just live a better lifestyle, the 7-Day Chair Yoga Meal Plan is your guide to bright health and energy. By including nutritious meals in your daily routine, you will not only improve your physical performance on the mat but also build a deeper sense of well-being that emanates from the inside.

So, if you're ready to go on a journey of holistic health and wellbeing, let's get started with the 7-Day Chair Yoga Meal Plan and experience the transformational power of feeding your body, mind, and spirit through mindful eating and yoga practice. Together, we'll build a lively, balanced, and joyful lifestyle that will help you achieve your best health and well-being.

Day 1: Energizing Start

Breakfast:

Overnight Oats with Almond Milk, Chia Seeds, Sliced Banana, and Almond Butter: Combine rolled oats, almond milk, chia seeds, sliced banana, and a dab of almond butter in a jar. Allow it to remain in the refrigerator overnight. In the morning, try this delectable and invigorating breakfast alternative.

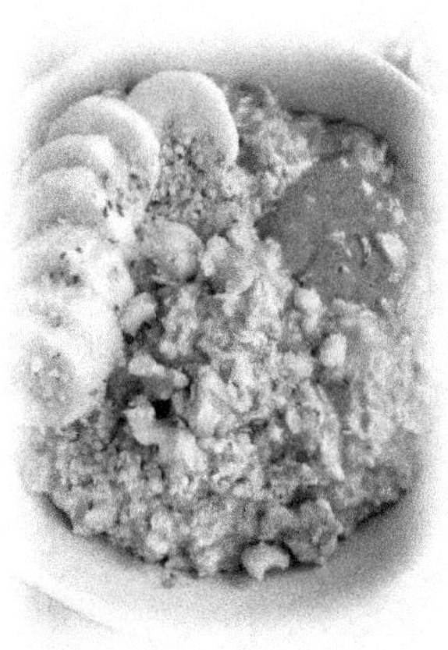

Overnight Oats with Almond Milk, Chia Seeds, Sliced Banana, and Almond Butter

Herbal Tea or Green Tea: Prepare a cup of herbal tea or green tea to go with your breakfast. These teas are refreshing and give a modest energy boost to get you started in the day.

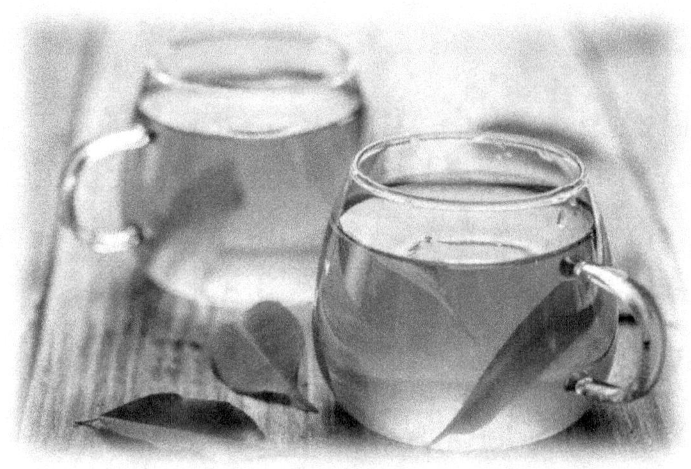

Green Tea

Lunch:

Spinach Salad with Grilled Chicken, Strawberries, Feta Cheese, and Balsamic Vinaigrette: Combine fresh spinach leaves, grilled chicken breast pieces, sliced strawberries, crumbled feta cheese, and a sprinkle of balsamic vinaigrette. This salad is loaded with nutrients and tastes to keep you full and invigorated.

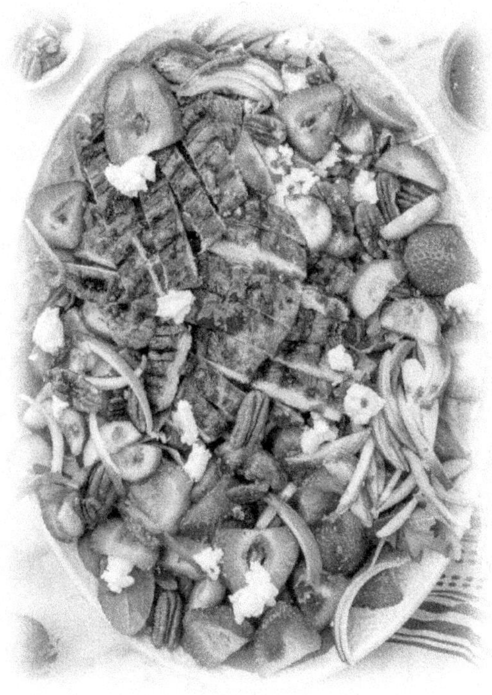

Spinach Salad with Grilled Chicken, Strawberries, Feta Cheese, and Balsamic Vinaigrette

Whole Grain Crackers with Hummus: For extra protein and fiber, serve whole grain crackers beside a hearty serving of hummus. This combo provides a pleasant and healthful lunch alternative.

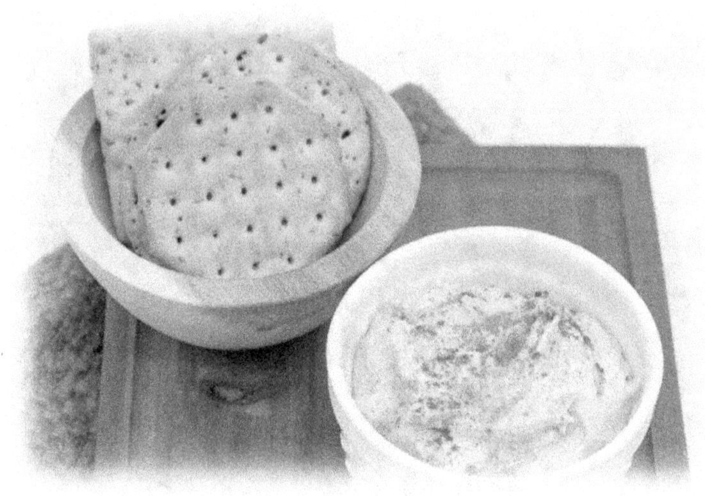

Whole Grain Crackers with Hummus

Snack:

Greek Yogurt with Mixed Berries and Honey: Top your Greek yogurt with a variety of berries (such as blueberries, raspberries, and blackberries) and drizzle with honey. This food is high in protein, vitamins, and antioxidants, which will keep you energized all day long.

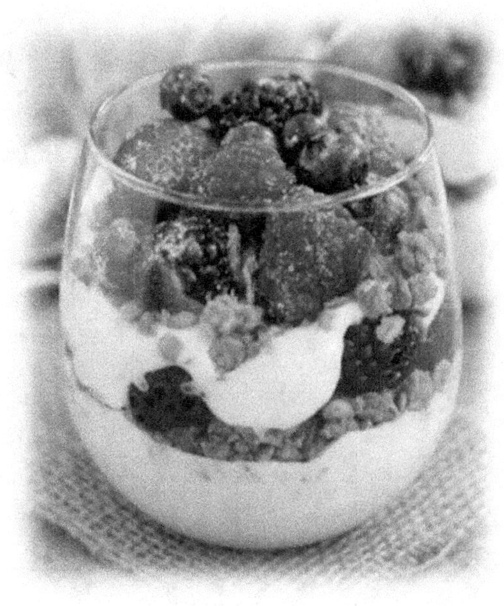

Greek Yogurt with Mixed Berries and Honey

Dinner:

Baked Salmon with Roasted Sweet Potatoes and Steamed Green Beans: For a wonderful meal, serve baked salmon fillets seasoned with herbs and lemon, alongside roasted sweet potato wedges and steamed green beans. This meal contains omega-3 fatty acids, vitamins, and minerals, making it a nutritious and delicious way to conclude the day.

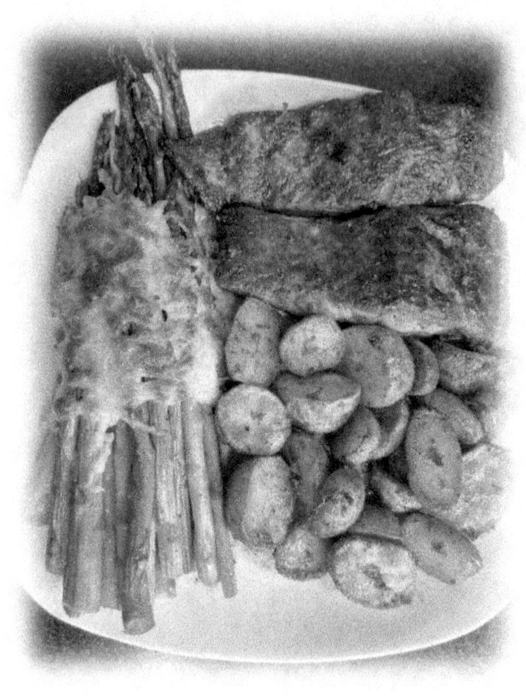

Baked Salmon with Roasted Sweet Potatoes and Steamed Green Beans

Day 2: Nourishing Nutrition

Breakfast:

Avocado Toast on Whole Grain Toast with Sliced Tomato and Everything Bagel Seasoning: Begin your morning with a slice of whole grain toast topped with mashed avocado, sliced tomato, and a sprinkle of everything bagel seasoning. This nutritious and tasty meal has healthy fats, fiber, and vitamins to help you get through the morning.

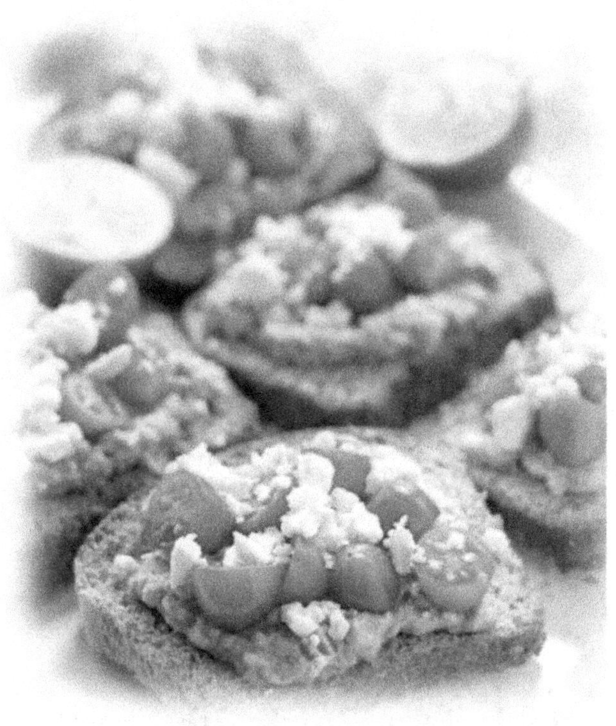

Avocado Toast on Whole Grain Toast with Sliced Tomato and Everything Bagel Seasoning

Herbal Tea or Matcha Latte: For a warm and comfortable beverage, have a cup of herbal tea or a matcha latte with your breakfast.

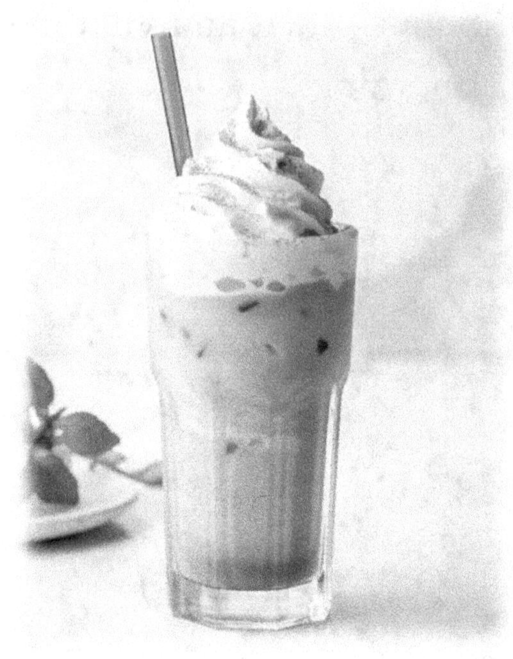

Matcha Latte

Lunch:

Quinoa & Black Bean Bowl with Roasted Vegetables and Avocado: For a substantial meal, combine cooked quinoa, black beans, roasted vegetables (such as bell peppers, zucchini, and onions), and sliced avocado. Drizzle with your favorite dressing or salsa for extra flavor.

Serve whole-grain tortilla chips with homemade guacamole for dipping. This combo offers a crunch and creamy texture to your meal, as well as healthful fats and fiber.

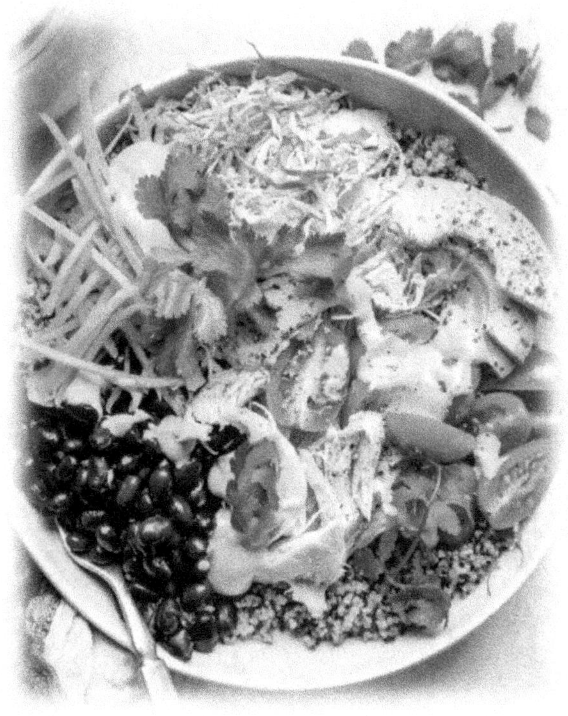

Quinoa & Black Bean Bowl with Roasted Vegetables and Avocado

Snack:

Sliced Apple with Peanut Butter: Combine a sliced apple with a spoonful of peanut butter for a filling and nutritious snack. The blend of sweet and savory tastes delivers an adequate balance of carbs, protein, and healthy fats.

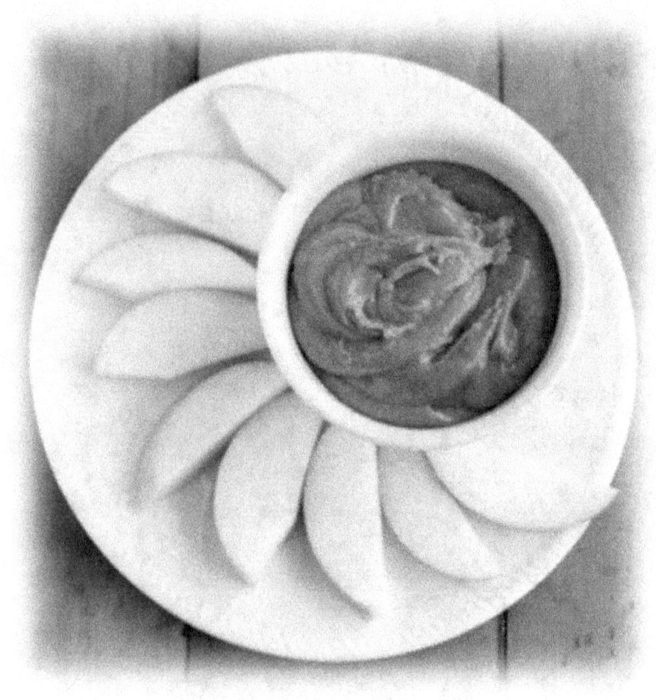

Sliced Apple with Peanut Butter

Dinner:
Turkey Meatballs with Whole Wheat Spaghetti and Marinara Sauce: Season turkey meatballs with herbs and spices, then serve over whole wheat spaghetti and marinara sauce. This nourishing and fulfilling supper choice is high in protein, fiber, and important minerals.

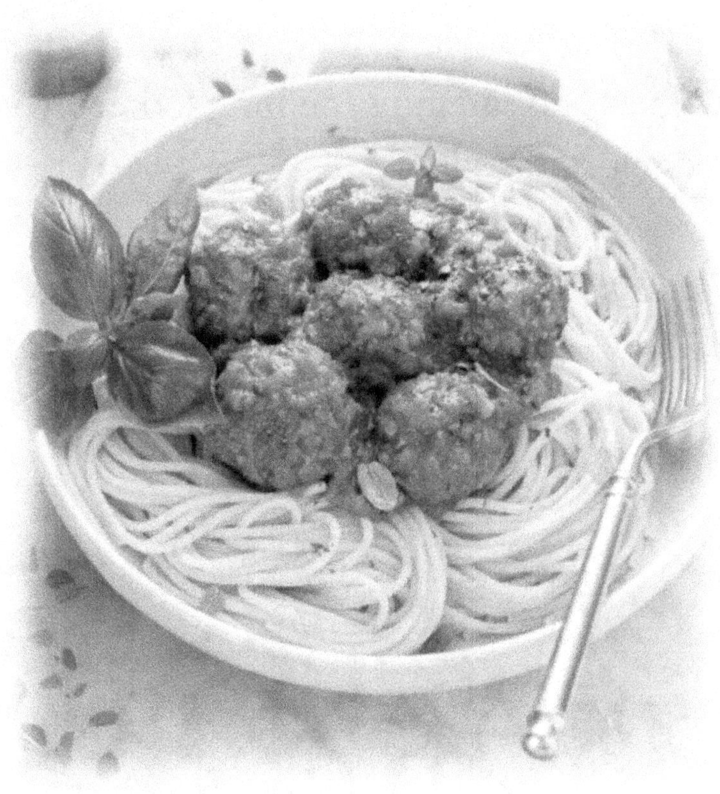

Turkey Meatballs with Whole Wheat Spaghetti and Marinara Sauce

Day 3: Balanced bliss.

Breakfast:

Greek yogurt parfait filled with granola, sliced peaches, and honey: Start your day with a delectable Greek yogurt parfait filled with granola, sliced peaches, and honey. This breakfast choice is high in protein, fiber, and vitamins, helping to keep you energized and satiated.

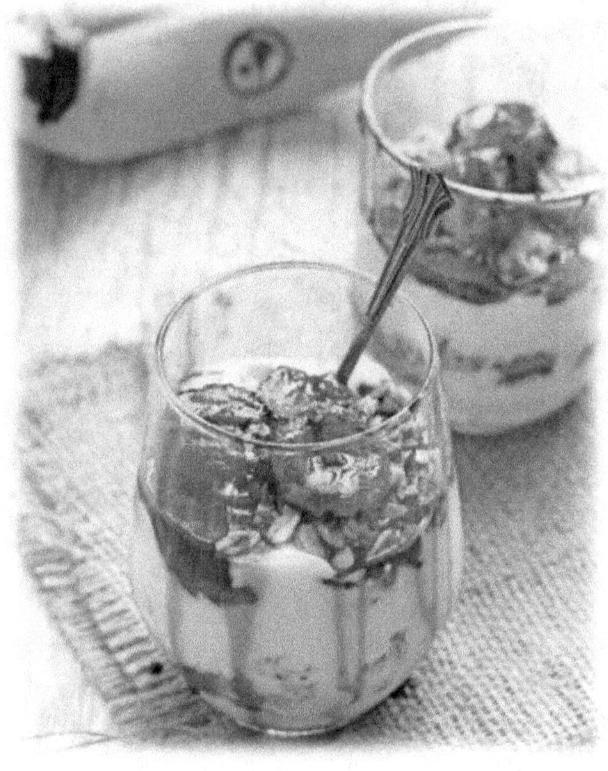

Greek yogurt parfait filled with granola, sliced peaches, and honey

Herbal tea or green tea: Drink a cup of herbal tea or green tea with your breakfast for a pleasant and calming beverage choice.

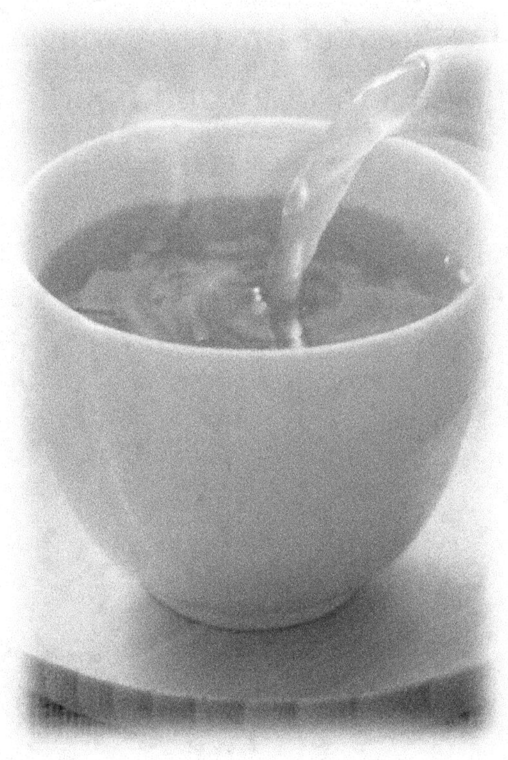

Herbal tea

Lunch:

Mediterranean Chickpea Salad with Cucumber, Cherry Tomatoes, Red Onion, Feta Cheese, and Lemon-Olive Oil Dressing: Make a colorful salad with chickpeas, cucumber, cherry tomatoes, red onion, crumbled feta cheese, and a tangy lemon-olive oil dressing. This salad is full of Mediterranean tastes and is high in protein, fiber, and antioxidants.

Serve whole grain pita bread as a side dish with creamy hummus for dipping. This combination enhances the texture and flavor of your meal while also providing added protein and fiber.

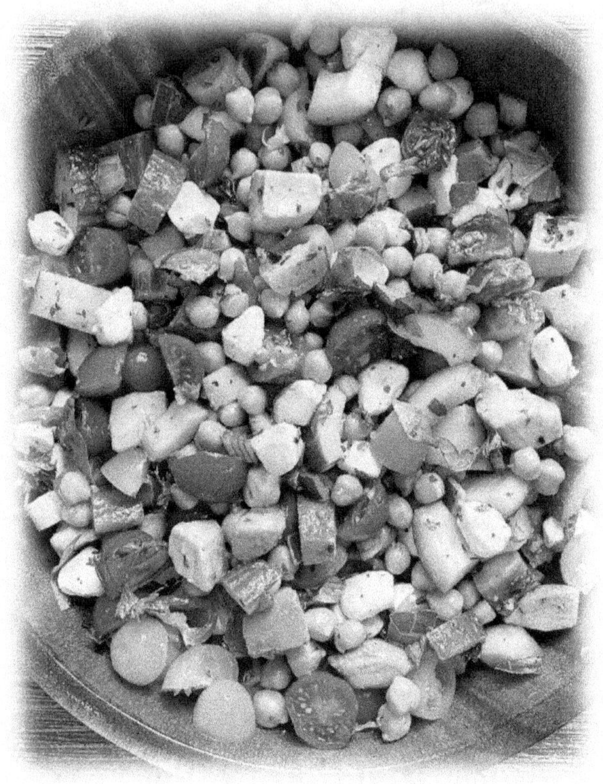

Mediterranean Chickpea Salad with Cucumber, Cherry Tomatoes, Red Onion, Feta Cheese, and Lemon-Olive Oil Dressing

Snack:

Carrot Sticks with Hummus: For a crisp and healthful snack, combine carrot sticks with hummus.

This snack gives a pleasant crunch as well as a vitamin and mineral boost, keeping you full and energized.

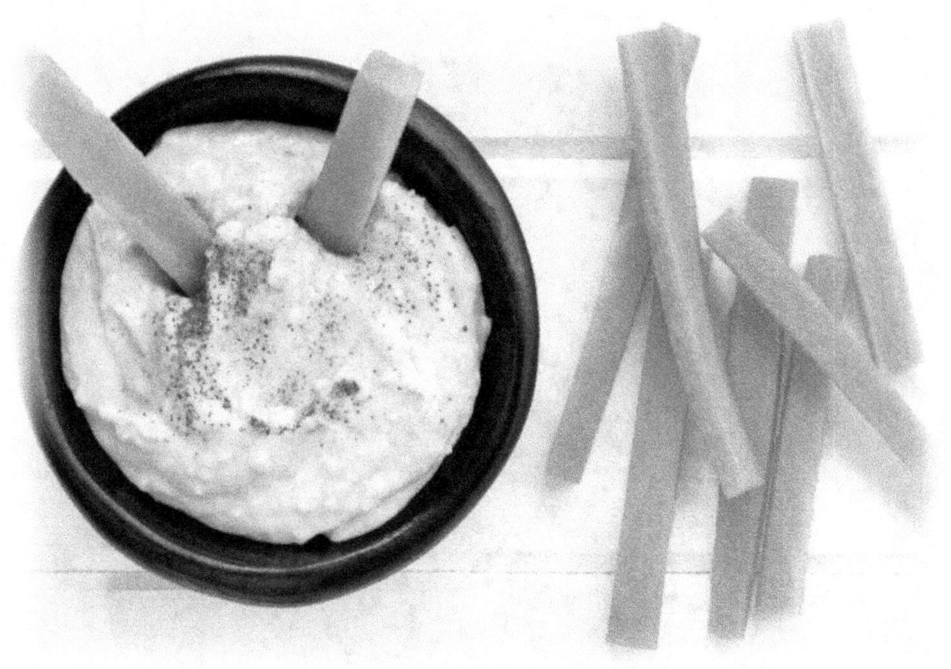

Carrot Sticks with Hummus

Dinner:
Stir-Fried Tofu with Mixed veggies in Teriyaki Sauce over Brown Rice: Make a tasty stir-fry with tofu, mixed veggies (such as broccoli, snap peas, and carrots), and teriyaki sauce, then serve over cooked

brown rice. This supper choice is high in plant-based protein, fiber, and important vitamins.

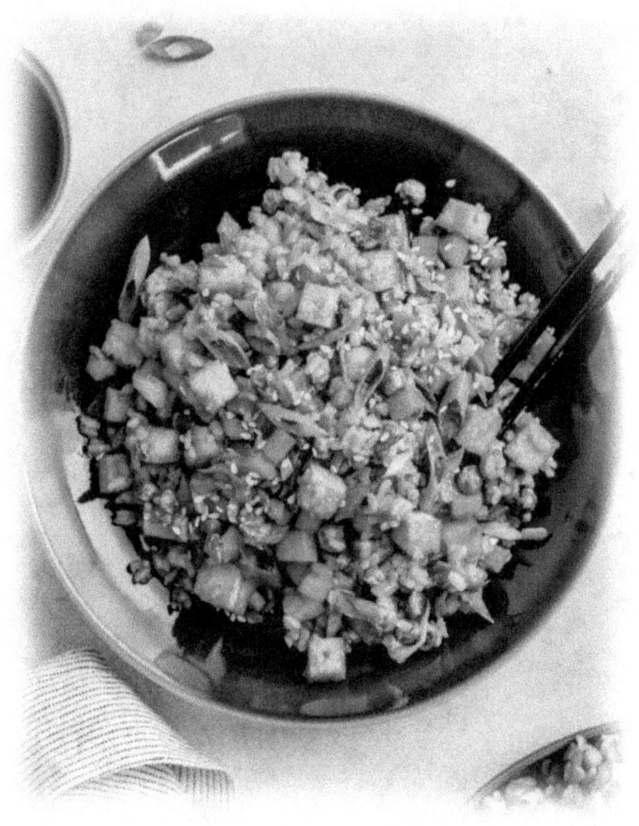

Stir-Fried Tofu with Mixed veggies in Teriyaki Sauce over Brown Rice

Day 4: Wholesome Delights.

Breakfast:

Veggie Omelette with Spinach, Bell Peppers, Onions, and Feta Cheese: Begin the day with a healthy veggie omelet cooked with eggs, spinach, diced bell peppers, onions, and crumbled feta cheese. This substantial breakfast choice is high in protein, vitamins, and minerals to keep you going throughout the morning.

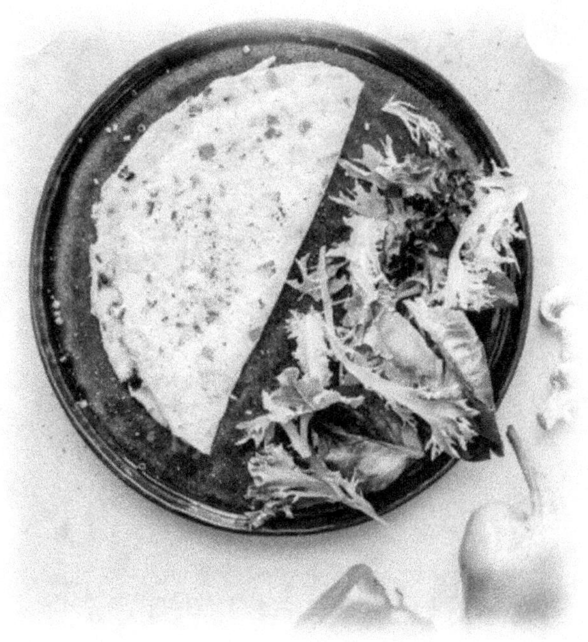

Veggie Omelette with Spinach, Bell Peppers, Onions, and Feta Cheese

Herbal Tea or Fruit-Infused Water: For a refreshing and energizing beverage, pair your breakfast with a cup of herbal tea or hydrating fruit-infused water.

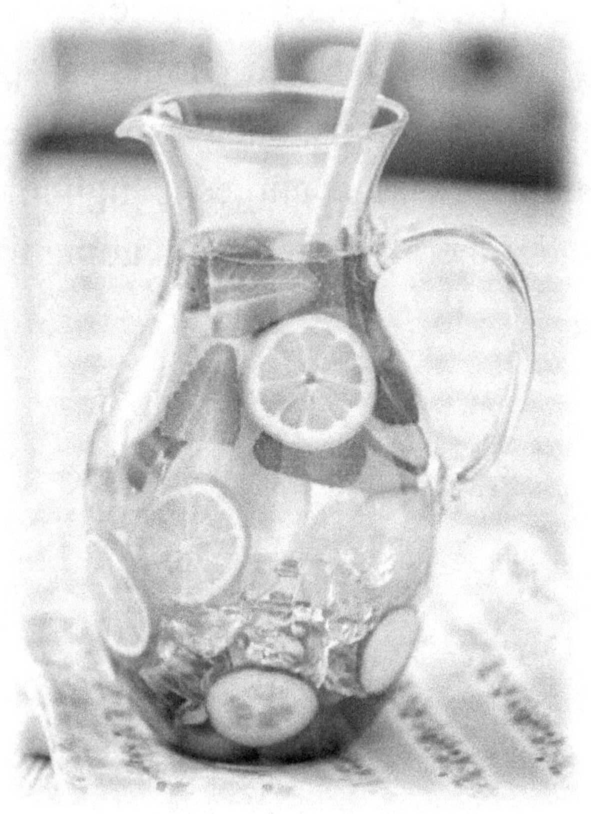

Fruit-Infused Water

Lunch:

Quinoa Salad with Roasted Vegetables, Chickpeas, and Lemon-Tahini sauce: Make a nutritious salad with cooked quinoa, roasted vegetables (including cauliflower, Brussels sprouts, and carrots), chickpeas, and a creamy lemon-tahini sauce. This salad is packed with fiber, protein, and healthy fats to keep you full and happy.

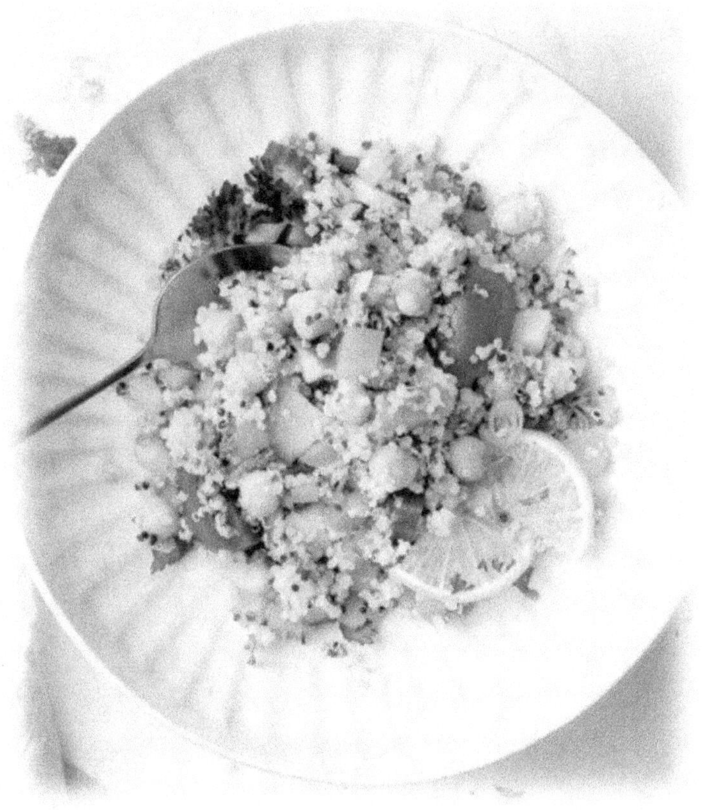

Quinoa Salad with Roasted Vegetables, Chickpeas, and Lemon-Tahini sauce

Whole Grain Crackers with Guacamole: Serve whole grain crackers alongside homemade guacamole for dipping. This combo adds crunch and creaminess to your meal while also providing critical minerals and healthy fats.

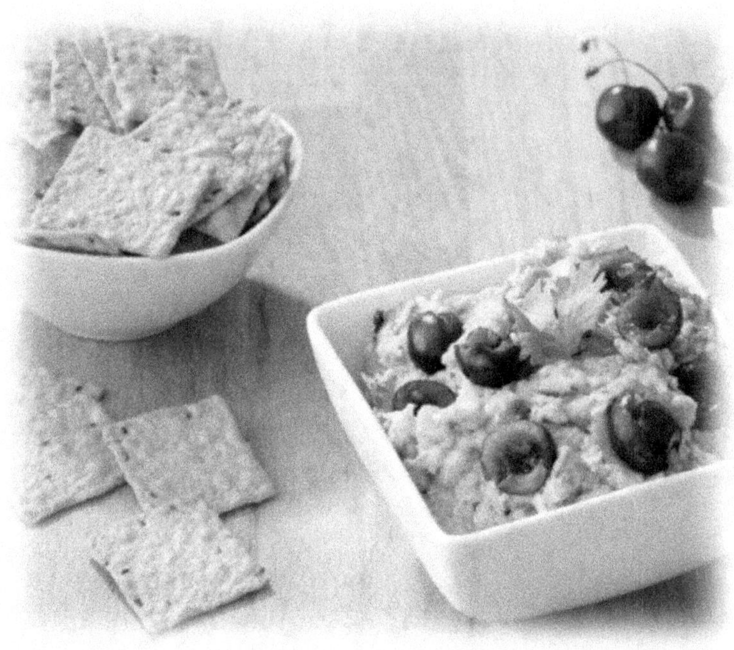

Snack:

Greek Yogurt with Sliced Strawberries and Almond Butter: For a pleasant and nutritious snack, top your Greek yogurt with sliced strawberries and a dab of almond butter. This combo contains protein, vitamins, and healthy fats to help you stay energetic throughout the day.

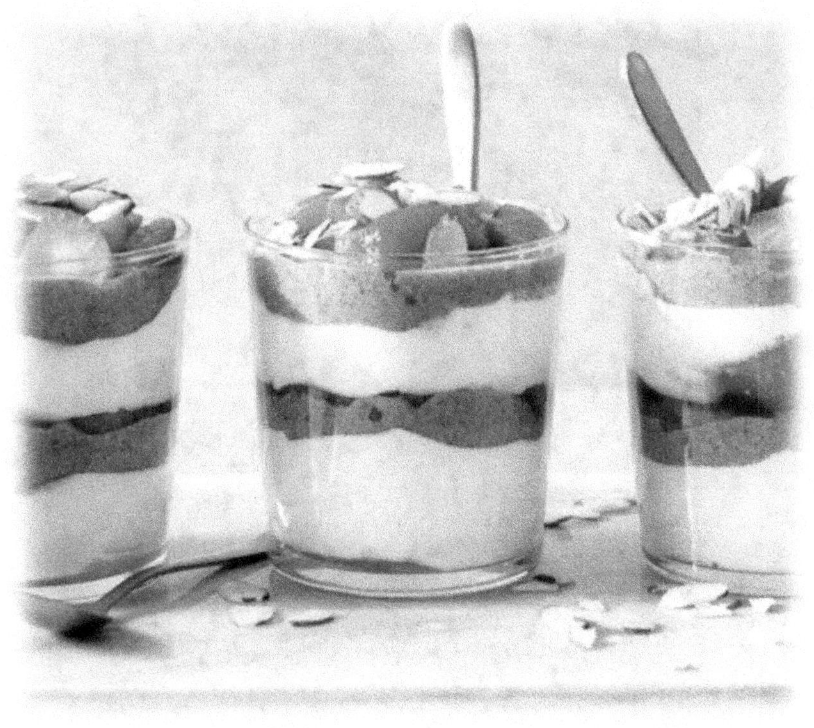

Greek Yogurt with Sliced Strawberries and Almond Butter

Dinner:

Baked Chicken Breast with Roasted Sweet Potatoes and Steamed Broccoli: For a delightful meal, serve baked chicken breast seasoned with herbs and spices over roasted sweet potato wedges and steamed broccoli florets. This meal is high in protein, fiber, and important minerals, nourishing your body while satisfying your taste senses.

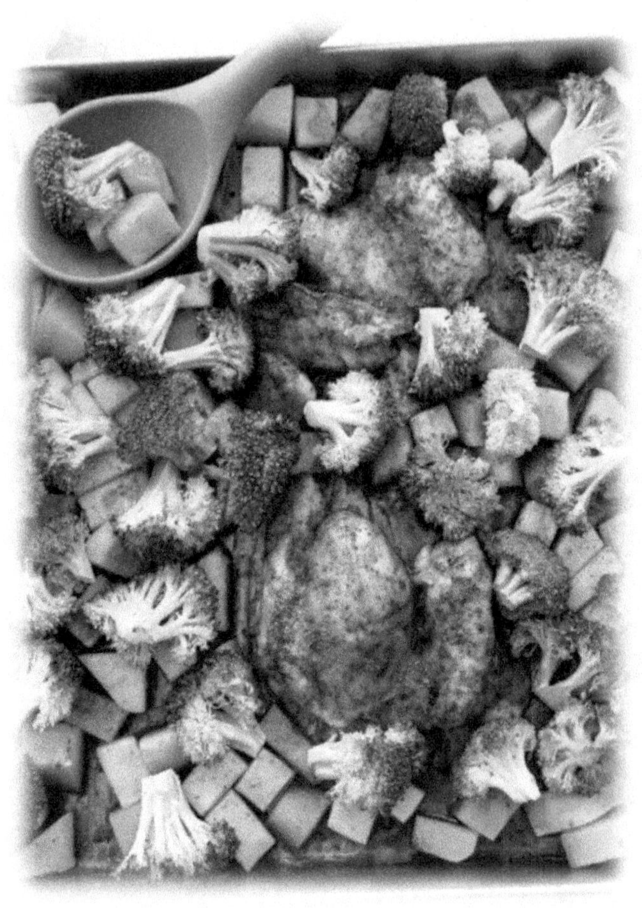

Baked Chicken Breast with Roasted Sweet Potatoes and Steamed Broccoli

Day 5: Flavored Feasts

Breakfast:

whole grain toast topped with smashed avocado, sliced hard-boiled egg: Start the day with a slice of whole grain toast topped with smashed avocado, sliced hard-boiled egg, and a sprinkling of everything bagel spice. This flavorful breakfast choice is high in protein, healthy fats, and fiber, which will keep you satiated and energized.

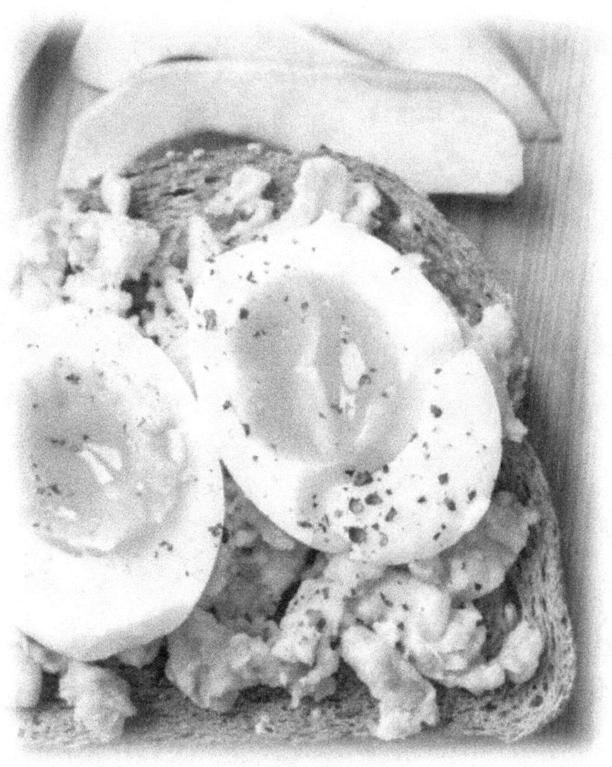

whole grain toast topped with smashed avocado, sliced hard-boiled egg

Herbal Tea or Fruit Smoothie: For a nutritious and hydrating beverage, pair your breakfast with a cup of herbal tea or a delightful fruit smoothie.

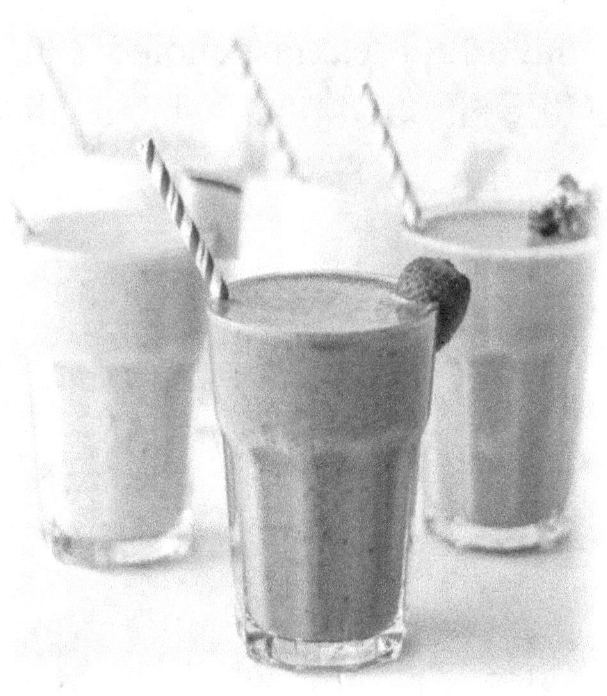

Fruit Smoothie

Lunch:

Lentil and Vegetable Soup with Whole Grain Bread: Make a hearty soup with lentils, mixed veggies (carrots, celery, and tomatoes), and aromatic herbs and spices. Serve the soup with a side of whole-grain bread to dip. This lunch choice is substantial, healthy, and ideal for a midday pick-up.

Enjoy a serving of mixed green salad with balsamic vinaigrette. This salad adds freshness and crunch to your lunch while also providing a nutritional boost.

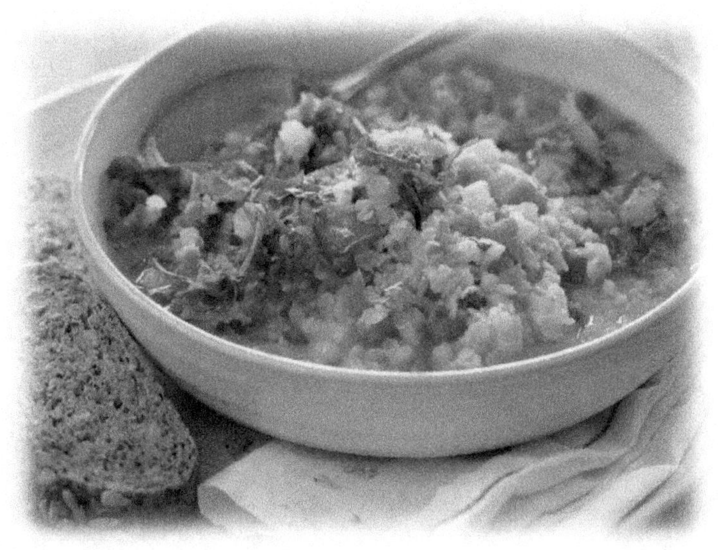

Lentil and Vegetable Soup with Whole Grain Bread

Snack:

Apple Slices with Almond Butter: Pair a sliced apple with a spoonful of almond butter for a filling and nutritious snack. The mix of sweet and nutty tastes delivers a wonderful balance of carbs, protein, and healthy fats to keep you motivated all day.

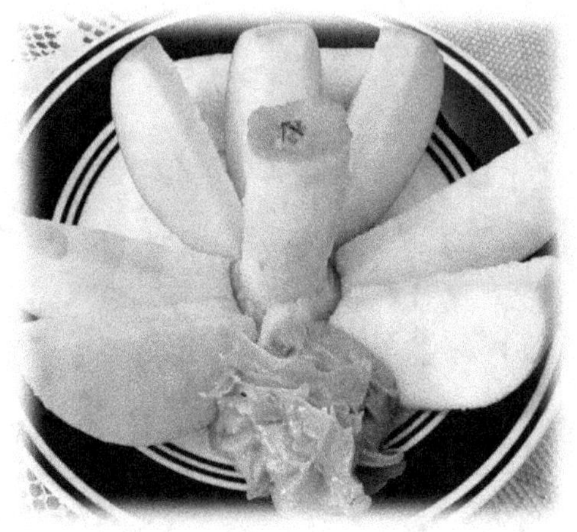

Apple Slices with Almond Butter

Dinner:

Grilled Salmon with Quinoa Pilaf and Steamed Asparagus: Make a tasty meal of grilled salmon fillets seasoned with herbs and lemon, served with quinoa pilaf and steamed asparagus spears. This meal is high in omega-3 fatty acids, protein, fiber, and important minerals, which fuel the body and promote overall health.

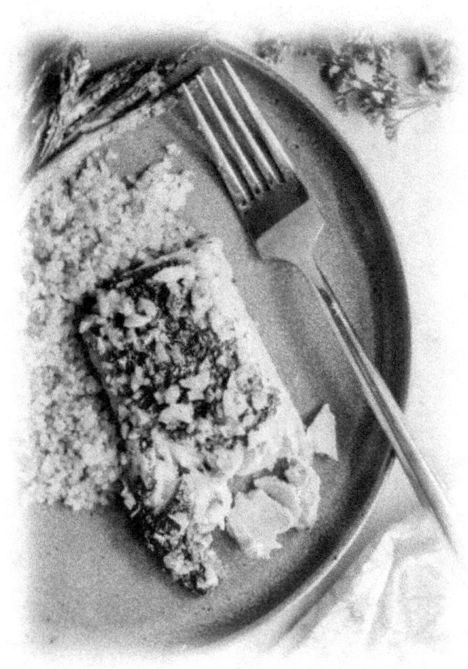

Grilled Salmon with Quinoa Pilaf and Steamed Asparagus

Day 6: Energizing Eats

Breakfast:
smoothie bowl prepared with mixed berries, spinach, Greek yogurt, and almond milk, topped with granola and chia seeds: Start your day with a refreshing smoothie bowl prepared with mixed berries, spinach, Greek yogurt, and almond milk, topped with granola and chia seeds. Top with granola and chia seeds for extra crunch and nutrients. This meal is high in vitamins, minerals, and antioxidants, making it an excellent way to start the day.

Drink a cup of herbal tea or a brilliant green juice with your breakfast for an extra burst of hydration and nutrients.

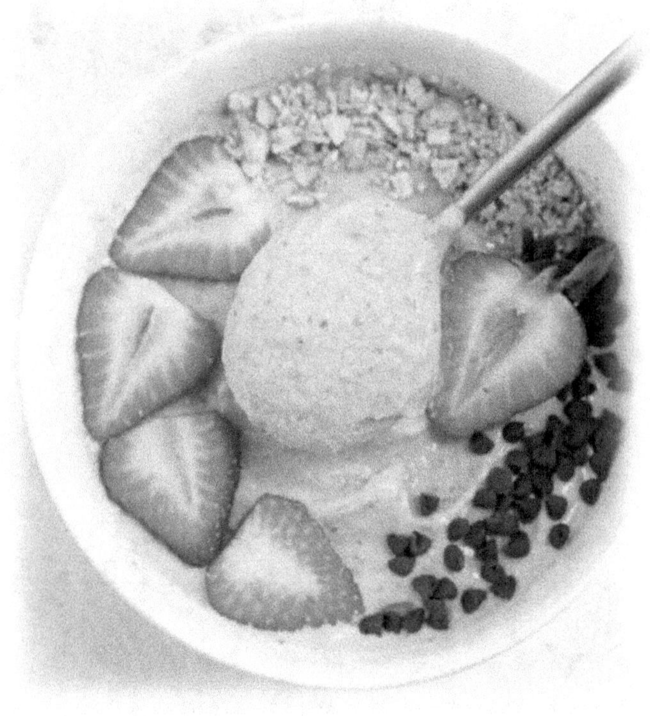

smoothie bowl prepared with mixed berries, spinach, Greek yogurt, and almond milk, topped with granola and chia seeds

Lunch:

Chickpea Salad Sandwich with Whole Grain Bread and Sliced Avocado: For a filling sandwich, combine mashed chickpeas, diced veggies (such as celery, red onion, and bell pepper), and a dollop of Greek yogurt or hummus. Serve on whole-grain toast with sliced avocado and lettuce. This lunch choice has enough protein, fiber, and healthy fats to keep you satisfied and energized.

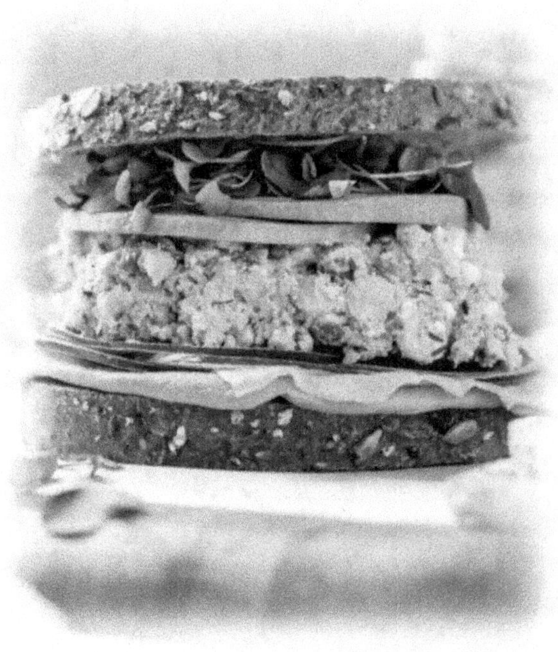

Chickpea Salad Sandwich with Whole Grain Bread and Sliced Avocado

Veggie Sticks with Hummus: Serve a side of veggie sticks (such as carrots, cucumber, and bell pepper) with creamy hummus to dip. This crispy and nutritious snack has a healthy blend of carbs, protein, and vitamins to keep you going all day.

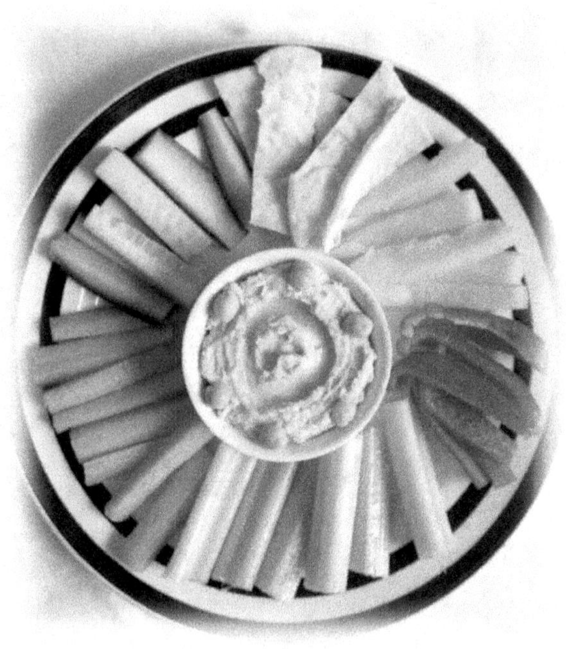

Veggie Sticks with Hummus

Snack:

Greek Yogurt with Mixed Berries and Honey: For a tasty and nutritious snack, top your Greek yogurt with mixed berries and a drizzle of honey. This mixture contains protein, antioxidants, and natural sweetness, which will fulfill your desires.

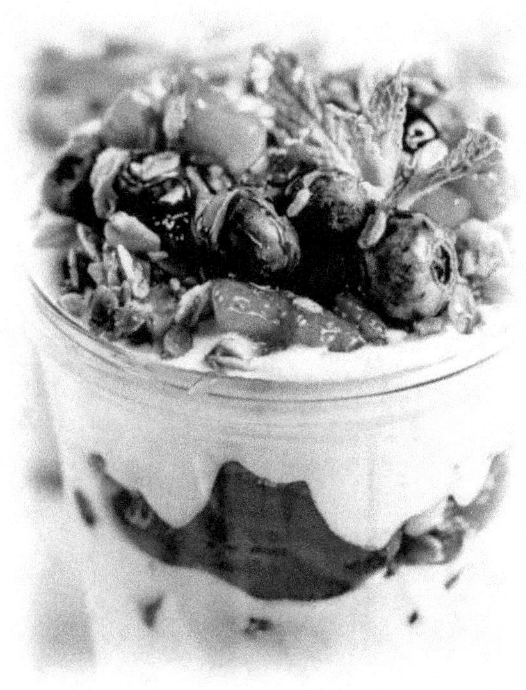

Greek Yogurt with Mixed Berries and Honey

Dinner:

Turkey Chili with Quinoa and Mixed Green Salad:
Make a hearty turkey chili using lean ground turkey, beans, tomatoes, and spices. Serve with cooked quinoa and a mixed green salad tossed with balsamic vinaigrette. This meal choice is high in protein, fiber, and important nutrients, which nourish your body and promote overall well-being.

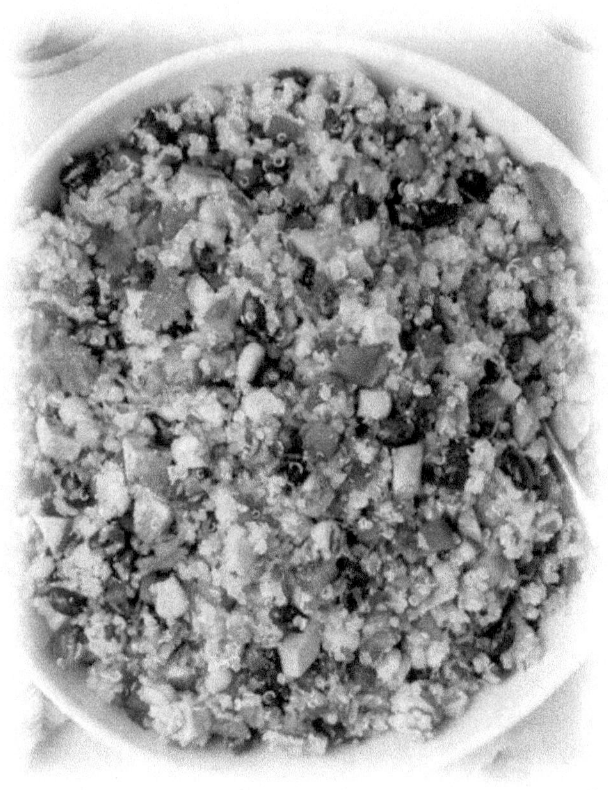

Turkey Chili with Quinoa and Mixed Green Salad

Day 7: Nourishing Nutrition

Breakfast:

Overnight Oats with Mixed Berries, Almonds, and Honey: Begin the day with a nutritious bowl of overnight oats cooked with rolled oats, almond milk, mixed berries, sliced almonds, and honey. Prepare the oats the night before for a quick and easy breakfast full of fiber, protein, and antioxidants.

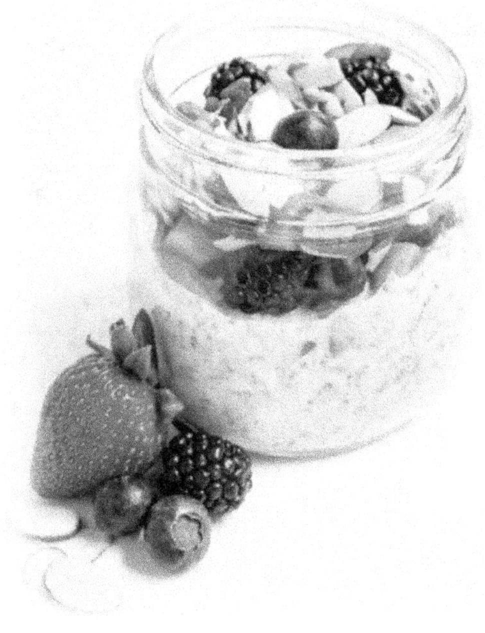

Overnight Oats with Mixed Berries, Almonds, and Honey

Herbal Tea or Warm Lemon Water: For hydration and a refreshing start to the day, pair your breakfast with a cup of herbal tea or a calming glass of warm lemon water.

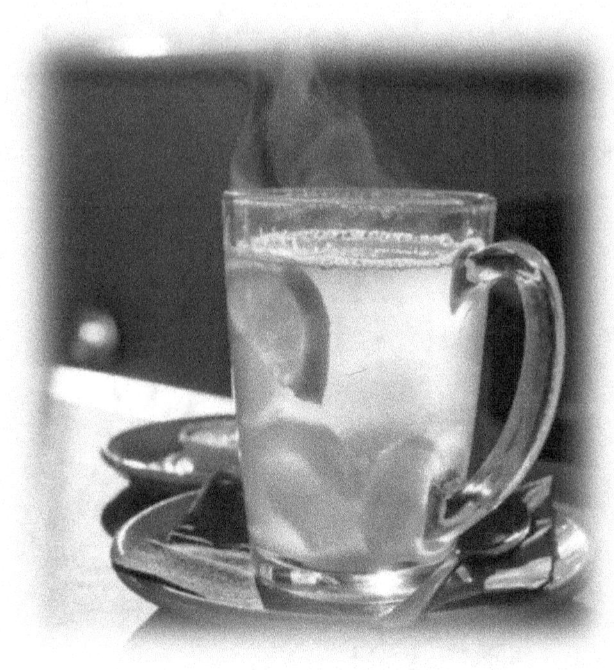

Warm Lemon Water

Lunch:

Roasted Vegetable and Quinoa Buddha Bowl with Tahini Dressing: Make a colorful Buddha bowl by combining roasted veggies (such as sweet potatoes, Brussels sprouts, and cauliflower), cooked quinoa, avocado slices, and tahini dressing. This lunch choice is high in fiber, protein, and healthy fats, which will keep you feeling full and energized.

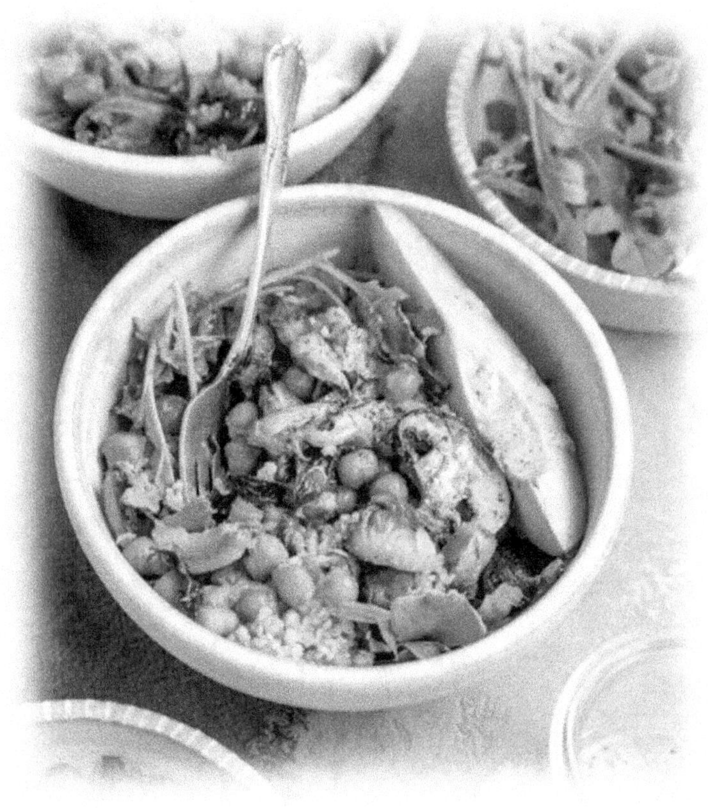

Roasted Vegetable and Quinoa Buddha Bowl with Tahini Dressing

Whole Grain Crackers with Cottage Cheese: Pair whole grain crackers with creamy cottage cheese for a crispy and protein-packed snack. This combo has a nice mix of carbs, protein, and nutrients, keeping you fed throughout the day.

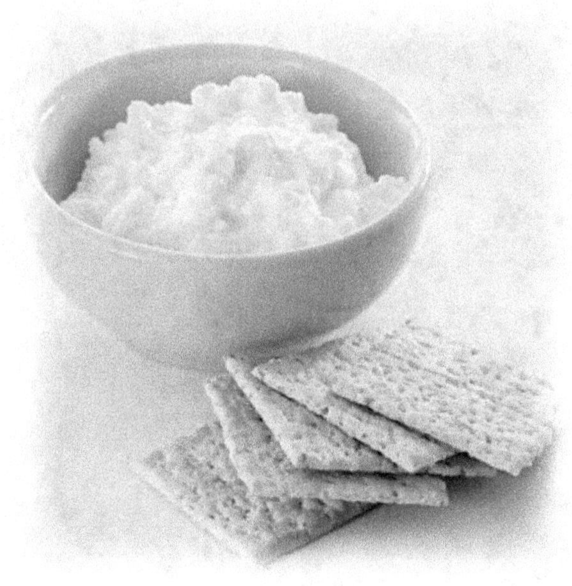

Whole Grain Crackers with Cottage Cheese

Snack:

Trail Mix with Dried Fruit, Nuts, and Seeds: For a filling and nutrient-dense snack, combine a handful of trail mix with dried fruit (such as raisins, apricots, and cranberries), mixed nuts (such as almonds, walnuts, and cashews), and seeds (such as pumpkin and sunflower seeds). Trail mix is a practical way to stay fueled on the road.

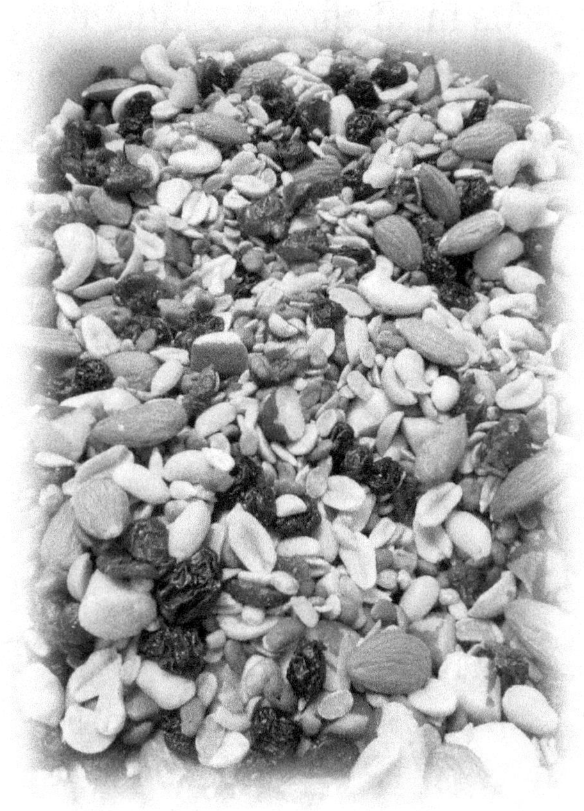

Trail Mix with Dried Fruit, Nuts, and Seeds

Dinner:

Grilled Veggie and Tofu Skewers with Quinoa Salad: Make delectable skewers with marinated tofu cubes and other veggies (such as bell peppers, zucchini, and cherry tomatoes) that are grilled to perfection. Serve with quinoa salad dressed with chopped cucumbers, tomatoes, parsley, and lemon vinaigrette. This meal choice is high in plant-based protein, fiber, and important nutrients, which fuel your body and promote overall health.

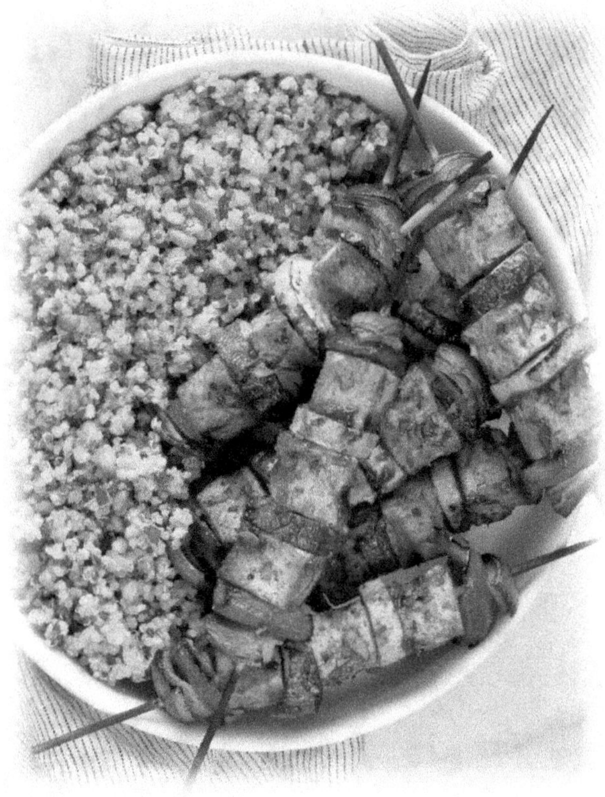

Grilled Veggie and Tofu Skewers with Quinoa Salad

Conclusion: Embrace Wellness with Chair Yoga

Congratulations on finishing "Chair Yoga for Seniors Over 60: Achieve Better Balance, Mobility, and

Flexibility with Simple, Quick, and Effective Yoga Exercises, Plus 7 Days of Recipes to Improve Your Health"! Throughout this book, we have looked at the transformational potential of chair yoga and how it may improve your physical and emotional health as you age.

From mild stretches to thoughtful movements, we've explored several chair yoga postures and practices that aim to enhance balance, flexibility, mobility, and general wellness. Whether you're new to yoga or an experienced practitioner, there's something for everyone on these pages.

We've also included a 7-day food plan full of nutritious and tasty meals to supplement your chair yoga practice. You can help your body achieve maximum health and vigor by feeding it nutritious meals.

As you continue your chair yoga adventure, keep in mind that consistency is crucial. Practice consistently, listen to your body, and respect your boundaries. Chair yoga is a practice of self-care and self-discovery, and each session allows you to connect with yourself on a deeper level.

Regardless of where you are on your wellness path, chair yoga may help you achieve increased balance, mobility, and flexibility. Incorporating these mild and accessible techniques into your daily routine will not only enhance your physical health, but will also foster a sense of calm, pleasure, and resilience in your life. Thank you for joining us on this path to greater health and wellness. May your chair yoga practice continue to motivate and inspire you for years to come.

I wish you good health, happiness, and peace.

[Anthony Howell]

Encouragement of Continued Practice and Growth

Congratulations on making it this far; I applaud you! As you've found throughout this book, chair yoga is a gentle but effective approach to enhance your physical and mental health, regardless of age or ability. As you continue to practice, here are some words of encouragement to help you improve and progress:

Consistency is Key: Remember that improvement in yoga, as in life, is frequently achieved via consistent practice. Even on days when you're weary or unmotivated, turning up on your mat and moving your body mindfully may make a big impact. Trust the process and understand that every practice, no matter how brief or basic, contributes to your total well-being.

Listen to Your Body: One of the most valuable benefits of yoga is learning to listen to your body's needs and knowledge. Pay attention to how each stance feels and make adjustments as needed to maintain your comfort and safety. Remember that yoga is about achieving balance and harmony within your own body and mind, not pushing yourself too hard.

Celebrate Your Progress: Take a minute to acknowledge how far you've gone in your yoga journey. Whether you've improved your balance, expanded your flexibility, or just discovered moments of quiet and relaxation, every tiny accomplishment is worth celebrating. Acknowledge your efforts and growth, no matter how small, and allow yourself to be proud of your achievements.

Stay Curious and Open-Minded: Yoga is a lifetime path of self-discovery and development. Approach your practice with curiosity and openness, ready to try new positions, methods, and ideas. Be kind to yourself as you traverse the ups and downs of your practice, and believe that each experience will provide useful lessons and insights.

Find Joy in the Journey: Most importantly, remember to enjoy your yoga practice. Whether you're moving through a series of postures, meditating in quiet, or simply breathing deeply, enjoy each moment and express thanks for the gift of movement and awareness. Allow your practice to bring you joy, inspiration, and a deeper connection to yourself and the world around you.

As you continue to practice chair yoga, may you discover strength, calm, and contentment both on and off the mat. Remember that you are capable of amazing development and transformation and that the journey is equally vital as the destination. Accept each step of the journey with bravery, curiosity, and an open heart.

Namaste.